FOOD AS MEDICINE

FOOD AS MEDICINE
a handbook of natural nutrition

Kirsten Hartvig ND, MNIMH, DipPhyt.

AEON

First published in 2023 by
Aeon Books

British Library Cataloguing in Publication Data

A C.I.P. for this book is available from the British Library

ISBN-13: 978-1-80-152-117-8

Typeset by Medlar Publishing Solutions Pvt Ltd, India

www.aeonbooks.co.uk

For Tessa

CONTENTS

INTRODUCTION   ix
  What is food?   xi
  Why do we eat?   xv

PART 1: NUTRITION

CHAPTER 1
The five basic nutrients   3

CHAPTER 2
Water: The most basic nutrient   5

CHAPTER 3
Standards   7

CHAPTER 4
Dietary deficiency   9

CHAPTER 5
Energy   11

CHAPTER 6
All about calories   13

CHAPTER 7
All about carbohydrates   21

CHAPTER 8
All about proteins   31

CHAPTER 9
All about fats   41

CHAPTER 10
All about vitamins   57

CHAPTER 11
All about major minerals and trace elements   89

CHAPTER 12
Antioxidants   123

PART 2: DIETETICS

CHAPTER 13
Naturopathic health principles   127

CHAPTER 14
Nutritional assessment   131

CHAPTER 15
Food as medicine   133

CHAPTER 16
What is a healthy diet?   137

CHAPTER 17
Diets and dieting   143

CHAPTER 18
Medicinal plant foods   161

CHAPTER 19
Politics and food production   181

REFERENCES   189

INTERNET SOURCES   193

ACKNOWLEDGEMENTS   195

AUTHOR BIOGRAPHY   197

INDEX   199

INTRODUCTION

When talking about using food as medicine, it is tempting to make up a list of foods and say what each of them are good for. And, as a herbalist and naturopath, I am often asked "have you got something for [insert complaint]?" But, as you will see on the following pages, health and disease are much more complex than that. Sometimes taking something away is more powerful and helpful than anything you could add, and any one food or herb or supplement can rarely cure a health problem that can have many different physical, emotional, mental, social, and spiritual aspects.

When you add to that the complexity of nutrition, nourishment, and nutrients, it is near impossible to work out what is good for what and why.

Then there's the case of whether you actually absorb any of the nutrients you consume. For example, iron absorption is inhibited by phytate and enhanced by vitamin C. Phytate, or phytic acid (aka hexaphosphate or IP6) is found in ungerminated seeds. It is a phosphate energy store providing the germinating seed the energy to grow. It is also found in animal, and therefore also human, cells where it is thought to act as a co-factor in DNA repair and in the production of the mRNA that is needed to make proteins. Humans and animals don't absorb phytate from their diet; they make their own! So, should you avoid phytates?

Phytates are found in the outer layers of some of the healthiest foods on the planet, where most vitamins and other micronutrients also occur in the highest concentrations. So why do people claim they are bad for you and call phytate an "antinutrient"? Because they say that phytate binds other nutrients (such as calcium, zinc, and iron) and prevents them from being absorbed. But that is not entirely true: although phytates inhibit absorption, it is only by a few percent. One study has shown that 13% of magnesium and 23% of zinc was absorbed in the presence of phytate in the same meal, as opposed to 30% without. Not a complete block, then, and absorption is dependent on many other factors such as stress and acidity, for example.

On the other hand, phytates also bring important health benefits to our gut biome and immune system: they inhibit the growth and spread of cancer cells; they help prevent absorption of heavy metals and help the body excrete them; they act as antioxidants by binding to minerals in the gut; they help protect against kidney stones by preventing calcification in body fluids; they interact with the natural gut bacteria to produce inositol, which helps the liver process fats, and lowers blood cholesterol and blood sugar.

Furthermore, foods high in phytate (aka phytic acid), such as beans, lentils, whole grains, nuts, and seeds, are also some of the most nutritious foods, high in micronutrients, antioxidants, and fibre, so it doesn't make sense to avoid it!

Or does it? People with malabsorption problems or at high risk of nutritional deficiencies or malnutrition should reduce their phytic acid intake by sprouting, soaking, fermenting, cooking, or baking phytate foods to increase the availability of their mineral content. Cooking phytate foods can increase their absorbability by 90%.

Eating phytate foods together with mineral-absorbing enhancers such as garlic and onion or foods high in vitamin C can also balance out the negative phytate effect while keeping its positive traits. So there is a strong case that rather than eating less phytate, you should eat more fresh fruit and onions and garlic, which have many other added health benefits!

This is just one example of the complexity of nutrition. It is my hope that by using this book as a reference, you will find your own way through this minefield and form your own opinion on what is good for you. Most of all, I hope it will empower you to enjoy eating plant foods and see them for what they are: the basis of all life on earth.

WHAT IS FOOD?

Food is made up of various substances, not all of which provide nutrition. Nutrients are substances that provide energy and raw material for the body. They enable living tissue to be built up and broken down.

There are five main categories of nutrients: protein, fat, carbohydrate, vitamins, and minerals. Besides nutrients, there may be other substances in food that have important effects on health, such as fibre and additives.

Whatever your dietary persuasion, it is important to remember that all the food we eat on earth can be traced back to plants. The issue is not what style of eating suits your particular type. Food is fundamentally much simpler than that: plants trap solar energy via photosynthesis and make it into a form of energy we can use. Green leaves are like solar panels, in this case converting light into carbs, which can then be used as they are, be gathered and stored as starch, or converted into fats and oils. It is a miraculous process where water drawn up from the earth meets carbon dioxide from the air and produces carbohydrates and oxygen. But that is another story we will explore more later.

Like people, plants also use protein to build structure. Proteins themselves are made from a combination of amino acids. Every structure and function of living organisms is made possible through the existence of amino acids. They are not only building blocks for proteins but also cell signalling molecules, and gene expression regulators. And some of them are responsible for maintenance, growth, reproduction, and immunity. Amino acids are also ultimately made by plants. They are compounds of carbon, hydrogen, oxygen, and nitrogen. They are the major nitrogen-containing compounds of plants. Plants are able to synthesise all the 20 amino acids used in the protein "alphabet" to create a multitude of proteins. The enzymes involved in the synthesis of the "essential" amino acids are normally located in leaves or roots and seeds.

Plants, fungi, microalgae, and microbiota also supply the micronutrients we need:

Vitamin D, for example, which, like carbohydrates, is created in response to exposure to sunlight but this time in animals, fungi, yeast, lichen, and planktonic microalgae at the base of the food chain. The presence of vitamin D in microalgae suggests that it may also be possible to find it in plants. Fur and feathers prevent sunlight from reaching the skin but in this case, sunlight interacts with the oil animals and birds produce to impregnate their fur and feathers. Sunlight interacts with the oil and produces vitamin D, which the birds and animals then ingest when they groom themselves.

Vitamin B12 is synthesised exclusively by aerobic and anaerobic fermenting soil microbiota (notably bacteria and archaea) that live in symbiotic relationships with plant roots, and it is also found naturally in fermented soya products (such as tempeh), algae and seaweeds (such as nori or laver). Although it is stored in the animal tissues we eat, it is not produced by animals.

The point I am making is that ALL the nutrients we need come from plants and microorganisms, so-called lower lifeforms at the bottom of the food chain. We may choose to let other species higher up the food chain do some of the digestion for us but the higher up the chain we are, the more vulnerable we become as only 10% of calories are passed on to the next link in the chain, but as much as 90% of the toxins.

In naturopathy and natural nutrition, we endeavour to eat food and nutrients as close to their original natural state as possible, as nature intended, and it therefore seems logical to cut out the middleman and do the digestion ourselves, right from the start. That way, it is much easier to be in control of what and how much we eat.

Were it only that simple, then many lifestyle problems would be easy to deal with. Imagine you only eat food direct from nature with as little preparation as possible, as people must have done back in the Stone Age, and as "primitive" people still do. Then your diet would consist mainly of the foods that are most readily available—greens, roots, fruits, and fungi. Nuts, seeds, and grains would be harder to come by—imagine if you had to grow, harvest, and prepare the grain from scratch for each piece of bread you were eating. Using vegetable oils would also be quite cumbersome if you had to pick, shell, and press the nuts and seeds yourself. Animal products would also be hard work—remember you'd have to feed the animals, as well as get them pregnant, milk your cow, and churn your butter. And how about the whole slaughtering process? Eggs might seem an easy option, but you'd have to feed the chickens through the winter too. With what? The grain you grew in the summer? But weren't you using that to make bread? Just imagine the effort that would go into making a simple cup of coffee with a pain-au-chocolat. Would you even know where to start? I wouldn't—imagine having to go to South America for the beans first, getting back in time to sow your wheat for the dough. Once you had all the ingredients, you'd have to roast the coffee beans, then work out how to make chocolate and pastry (you'd need a cow or a coconut too to get the fat to mix in the layers). I suspect you'd need some sugar cane or turnip too and find out how to refine it into a usable form.

To make it as easy as possible, let's presume you'd want your coffee black, saving the milk to make the fat for the pastry. When you'd got all the ingredients, you'd be faced with the enormity of the task it is to make pastry for the pain-au-chocolat! I don't know if you've ever tried it? It takes all day, as well as considerable skill!

Putting the oven on, now where is your source of heat? A bonfire underneath? Remember, there were no electricity supply or power stations, oil or gas in Palaeolithic times.

So, of course I'm not suggesting we go back to times without modern creature comforts or coffee and pain-au-chocolat. What I would like to suggest is that we don't copy the humans that roamed the earth in those days—but rather put the emphasis on the essential lifeforms that were there then and had been there for millions of years already, not only surviving but also forming the basis for all other lifeforms: plants and microorganisms!

If you want to eat a paleo diet, therefore, eat plants and lichens, seaweeds and algae. There is no real and nutritionally meaningful difference between eating a fish, bird or animal that has absorbed the micronutrients we need from plants and microorganisms in their tissues and thus passing them onto us; or cutting out the middleman and eating the nutrients directly as a food or supplement. So why don't we?

WHY DO WE EAT?

Have you ever asked yourself that question? Everyone knows that we eat to satisfy hunger and nourish the body, but if it were that simple, our diet could be very simple and unrefined too. But think of your relationships—business or personal—and how important it can be to initiate or maintain relationships over food and drinks. Or how you can demonstrate the nature and extent of your relationships by your food choices...

Food also provides a focus for communal activities. We serve food to express love and caring, to symbolise emotional experiences, to express moral sentiments and individuality, and to separate ourselves from a group, or demonstrate we belong to a group!

When life is challenging, we eat to cope with psychological and emotional stress, or we eat to reward or punish ourselves, and certain meals and foods are served to signify social status, to bolster self-esteem and gain recognition. Food or denial of food can also be used to wield political or economic power, with the scarcity of popular or vital foods being used to persuade populations in one direction or the other. In that sense, food can be used to represent wealth and security too.

The point is, that since there are so many good and bad reasons why people eat, dieting and eating for health is much more complex than it would seem on the surface.

The real question is: who is in charge? If it is you, then a good starting point is to get to know what the foods you eat are made of, and what the consequences of excess and deficiency of any particular nutrient in your diet might be. This will enable you to choose foods to remedy nutritional deficiencies and imbalances, and to develop dietary strategies to help in the management of common health problems.

PART 1

NUTRITION

CHAPTER 1

The five basic nutrients

To maintain normal function, the body requires adequate intakes of the following:

1. Water—the most important basic nutrient! Drinking enough water is as important as eating enough good food. The body needs water to maintain blood flow, to produce secretions, and to perform metabolic reactions.
2. Energy—energy for life comes from the sugars, starches, and oils that are made by plants from sunlight, air, and water. These are then eaten by us directly as plant-based foods, or indirectly as animal-based foods.
3. Vitamins—vitamins are essential chemical co-workers that help cellular enzymes to regulate metabolic reactions.
4. Minerals—minerals are used to facilitate various electrical and chemical processes.
5. Proteins—these are the "building blocks" from which muscles, blood, hormones, and new tissues are made by the body.

CHAPTER 2

Water: The most basic nutrient

Increasing your daily water intake can have a profound effect on your health and wellbeing. Water—without anything added—can be more powerful than any medication in promoting health and treating disease. But please note that tea, coffee, herb tea, juice, or any other manufactured beverages do not count as water.

Water makes up over two thirds of the human body. Dehydration happens when the body loses more fluid than is taken in. It is a surprisingly common problem even though everyone knows that water is vital for all life on earth. The human body is dependent on water for the blood to circulate and bring nutrients to all the 30 trillion cells we consist of. It is equally important for the removal of waste and toxins from the tissues and organs, and to help the kidneys function properly.

Water is also a vital part of our temperature control system as the process of perspiration places a layer of water on the entire surface of the body, thereby cooling the whole system down.

Common causes of dehydration include not drinking enough fluid to replace what is used. Climate and exercise can contribute, as can illness, fever, vomiting, and diarrhoea.

It is commonly thought that manmade drinks are superior to pure natural water, but every addition of constituents adds a burden on the body's processing and filtering system. Drinks containing sugar and caffeine may cause dehydration, as do many herbs and medications—despite their medicinal value.

Dehydration eventually leads to loss of function of the body's vital organs, including the brain! Because we sometimes forget the vital importance of water, we often misinterpret thirst and signs of dehydration and think we need food and medication when the problem could be solved by increasing our water intake.

Silencing the signals of water shortages leads to chronic dehydration, which can have serious consequences, including headache, dizziness, heat exhaustion, tiredness, hypertension, sore throat, asthma and allergies, gastric ulcers and gastrointestinal irritation, constipation, urinary tract infections, kidney problems, kidney stones, skin problems, muscle damage, and rheumatic complaints. If left untreated, severe dehydration can cause fits, brain damage, and death.

Babies and infants, athletes, older people, people with long-term health problems such as diabetes or alcoholism are most at risk from dehydration.

Like any other deficiency, the most efficient cure for dehydration is to supply the missing ingredient! Rehydration has an immediate and powerful effect because disturbance in the body's water metabolism influences everything from hormone balance to enzymes and neurotransmitter function. The supply of nutrients, and removal of toxins and waste from every organ, system and cell depends on an adequate supply of water.

Drinking enough pure water is thus an important part of any diet regime, but it is also possible to become overhydrated, especially while exercising, sweating, and drinking lots of water over a short period of time. The condition is called hyponatremia and can affect athletes who lose sodium through sweating and at the same time dilute the sodium content in their bloodstream by drinking large amounts of water. Symptoms include nausea, vomiting, and headache.

CHAPTER 3

Standards

The question "how much do I need to eat of each nutrient?" sounds simple but is difficult to answer. Orthodox nutrition is based on research that finds out what people eat, analyses the food eaten into component nutrients and compares the amounts of those nutrients with standard values:

Recommended Dietary or Daily Intakes (RDI): The RDI is the average daily intake level of a particular nutrient that is likely to meet the nutrient requirements of 97–98% of healthy individuals in a particular life stage or gender group.

Recommended Dietary Allowance (RDA): The RDAs are the level of intake of essential nutrients that, on the basis of scientific knowledge, are judged to be adequate to meet the known nutrient needs of practically all healthy people.

Dietary Reference Values (DRVs): DRVs are a series of estimates of the energy and nutritional requirements of different groups of healthy people in the population. They are not recommendations or goals for individuals.

Estimated Average Requirements (EARs): The EAR is an estimate of the average requirement of energy, or a nutrient needed by a group of people (ie approximately 50% of people will require less, and 50% will require more).

Reference Nutrient Intakes (RNIs): The RNI is the amount of a nutrient that is enough to ensure that the needs of nearly all in a group (97.5%) are being met.

Lower Reference Nutrient Intakes (LRNIs): The LRNI is the amount of a nutrient that is enough for only a small number of people in a group who have low requirements (2.5%), that is the majority need more.

Safe Intake: The Safe Intake is used where there is insufficient evidence to set an EAR, RNI or LRNI. The Safe Intake is the amount judged to be enough for almost everyone, but below a level that could have undesirable effects.

However, the validity of these standards is open to question as they are only estimates. They have wide inbuilt safety margins and are calculated for a standard population. They may thus over- or under-estimate the needs of individuals. In many cases, RDAs are little better than educated guesses, as illustrated by the very large variations in values for the same nutrient recommended in different countries. On the whole, British RDAs tend to be lower than those used in the USA, although the recommended intakes for several nutrients have been reduced by the American Food and Drug Administration.

The introduction of DRVs in the UK was an attempt to take individual variation into account but apply only to the intake of energy, protein, vitamins, and minerals. Specific requirements for fats, sugars, and starches are not defined, although the proportions of these in the diet may also affect health.

The tables in this book relate the nutrient contents of different foods to the EAR (RDA).

CHAPTER 4

Dietary deficiency

Since there is no widely accepted definition of optimum health, it is hard to decide how much protein or vitamin C or calcium a person needs to eat to avoid poor health. Moreover, most people will remain well eating far less than the "recommended amounts" of many nutrients, and that makes it difficult to assess the adequacy of any individual's diet.

The situation is further complicated by the fact that absorption of some nutrients is far from complete in normal humans. More than 90% of the proteins, fats, and carbohydrates in food are digested and absorbed but only about 15% of the iron gets into the body—and even that figure depends on other factors such as other dietary constituents and the form in which the iron occurs in the food.

In other words, the fact that the daily intake of a nutrient may fall below recommended levels is not on its own indicative of a deficiency risk.

Deficiency refers to a state characterised by adverse symptoms; a lower than recommended consumption or even a lower-than-average blood level of a nutrient will not necessarily cause ill-health. In many instances, the body seems able to adapt to low levels of nutrient intake by increasing the efficiency of absorption and reducing excretion.

CHAPTER 5

Energy

Food provides energy for muscular work and general body maintenance, and the body must meet its energy requirements before making use of other nutrients, but this is easily done if enough food is eaten.

Energy is measured in kilocalories (kcal) or joules (j). A calorie is a unit of heat energy, technically defined as "the energy needed to raise the temperature of one gram of water by one degree centigrade".

In the body, the process of metabolism converts the calories contained in food into the energy we need to live. As even small amounts of food can contain thousands of calories of energy, it has become standard practice to express food energy in terms of kilocalories (kcal), where 1 kilocalorie = 1000 calories.

Energy provided by macronutrients

1 gram carbohydrate	=	4 kcal
1 gram protein	=	4 kcal
1 gram fat	=	9 kcal
1 gram alcohol	=	7 kcal

Fat is much more calorie dense than protein or carbohydrate because it is designed for the compact storage of energy. This is a problem if you want to lose weight, as one kilo of body fat contains 9000 kcal and provides about 4–5 days of energy, so losing 10 kg can easily take a couple of months even if you don't eat anything at all. The upside is that if you are a bird and want to fly from one end of the earth to the other, as many of them do twice a year, your body fat provides plenty of energy without too much weight to carry.

CHAPTER 6

All about calories

It is possible, using charts and tables, to work out exactly how many calories we need for our age, height, and activity level. However, the bottom line is simple: we need as many as we use! Children use calories for growth and are usually very active; but they are also small, so they need fewer calories than adults overall. Older people are generally less active, so they also need fewer calories. Pregnant and nursing mothers need more calories than average women because they have two mouths to feed. Overweight bodies use up more energy than non-overweight bodies because they carry around extra weight.

If we eat more calories than we need, the extra energy released from food is converted into fat and stored for later use. If we don't use up our fat stores, we become overweight. As we shall see in more detail later, once fat cells have been created, they remain, although they can be emptied of fat. The problem with childhood obesity is that you will always have more fat cells waiting to be filled.

Calories and appetite

The appetite is our natural in-built calorie counter that ensures we take in enough energy to fuel our daily activities. It makes us feel hungry when we need energy, and full when we've eaten enough. If we eat healthy food, the appetite does the calorie counting automatically. So, to take a major step toward maintaining a healthy weight, all we need to do is learn to pay attention to the signals that our bodies give us about what we need, rather than to what our eyes tell us we want.

Empty calories

For most of us, empty calories for a substantial part of our daily diet, making it hard for us to hear the quiet voice of a healthy appetite.

A typical empty-calorie diet

Breakfast	White buttered toast with jam, coffee with milk and sugar
Morning snack	Chocolate bar, coffee with milk and sugar
Lunch	Burger in a white bun with chips, and a soda
Afternoon snack	Cake or biscuits, tea with milk and sugar
Dinner	An aperitif with some crisps followed by a processed food meal accompanied by another drink or two.

Although this diet provides plenty of calories, it is high in saturated fat and refined carbohydrates, and it contains little useful nourishment or micronutrients. Excess saturated fat leads to the formation of dangerous fatty deposits in the blood vessels; excess refined carbohydrate disrupts energy levels by upsetting the blood sugar balance; and calories derived from alcohol place strain on the liver.

Processed foods that combine carbs with fats (a cream cake, for example) are popular because they produce a feeling of immediate satisfaction. The brain is happy because it has been given plenty of resources to cope with a sudden stress situation—the sugar rush provides a feeling of being able to cope with anything—while the body is satisfied with the immediate fat reserves.

However, these feelings don't last because the calories are not accompanied by other nutrients the body needs, and the blood sugar soon falls as the release of extra insulin speeds up its uptake into body cells and conversion into more body fat. In fact, it only takes 4 hours for any excess calories to be deposited as body fat and thus not immediately available for energy, but that's another story…

As a result, we are tempted to eat more empty calories and risk being trapped in a vicious circle of poor nutrition and increasing weight. More people pig out on chocolate biscuits than on carrots, but even if you were to binge on carrots, the damage in terms of calories would be minimal: four chocolate biscuits contain over 500 kcal, while four carrots contain just 35 kcal. Whether you are interested in slimming, or simply want to maintain a healthy weight, the vital step is to make the change from chocolate biscuits to carrots—from calorie-dense, micronutrient-deficient empty calories to a micronutrient-rich, high-quality calorie diet of unprocessed foods.

Quality calories

The calories contained in almost any unprocessed food are well-balanced in packages that make it harder to overeat. This is because the act of processing takes the nutrients out of their natural context and make them more easily available. Think of eating unshelled nuts as opposed to nut butter. If you have to shell each nut first, it takes much longer to eat the same amount of calories as you would get in a spoonful of nut butter.

Eating more unprocessed foots will improve the nutritional quality of your diet and make it easier to keep up your energy levels with fewer calories overall. Simply by basing your diet on unprocessed foods, you will become healthier and find it easier to maintain an optimum weight in the long term.

The benefit of eating quality calories from unprocessed foods is that they are

– High in fibre and complex carbs

– High in polyunsaturates and essential fatty acids

– A rich and balanced source of protein and essential amino acids

– Rich in all important minerals and trace elements

– High in natural antioxidants

– Low in cholesterol

– Low in "bad fats"

– Low in refined carbs

– Free from harmful additives.

The proteins, carbohydrates, fibre, fats, vitamins, minerals, trace elements, and phytochemicals contained within the calories we eat give us energy to perform our daily tasks, and also help to prevent illness and promote healing. If you cut down on calories to lose weight, it is crucial that the food you eat has the right balance of nutrients. Choosing low-calorie unprocessed foods ensures that your dietary needs are met while you are losing weight.

Obesity and eating disorders

Obesity means excess body fat, and is usually caused by a mixture of poor eating habits, lack of health education, metabolic disorders, depression, genetic predisposition, childhood diet, and other social factors. It is also associated with a number of serious medical conditions, including coronary heart disease and cancer. One in six American children are overweight, and it is estimated that the obesity epidemic costs Americans $260 billion a year in treatment.

People who are overweight clearly eat more calories than they use and, because they have more fat cells to feed, they have an altered sensitivity to hunger and fullness. This may also be linked to reduced psychological resistance to sensory stimuli such as sight, smell, and taste. Watching television is strongly associated with obesity because it provides strong sensory stimuli while promoting a sedentary lifestyle and lowering metabolic rate. This combination induces a trance-like state that makes it difficult to get up from the sofa and do something active.

To complicate matters, fat cells seem to have been designed to make dieting difficult. If, as a result of calorie restriction, fat cells become smaller, they send increasingly powerful signals to the brain asking to be fed, resulting in an overpowering urge to eat. The larger number of fat cells, the stronger the urge, which explains why when fat people, who have more fat cells, follow severe diets, which shrink their fat cells rapidly, they frequently suffer a "rebound" effect from dieting and put on more weight after the diet than they lost by following it. In fact, studies suggest that only five per cent of obese people are able to slim down at all and maintain an "ideal" body weight in the long term, which explains the continued proliferation of books on diet and dieting. A wise physician once said that the more treatments that are available for a disease, the less likely it is that any of them actually work.

Maximising sustainable weight loss involves losing weight slowly (between 250–500g per week). If you want to lose a pound a week, you must use up 500 calories more than you eat each day, which can be achieved by taking half an hour of aerobic exercise daily, or by exchanging bread and biscuits with raw vegetables while keeping your energy use the same.

A regular meal pattern with little or no snacking makes it easier to refrain from binge eating, and food containing plenty of fibre helps to keep the digestive system occupied. Also ensure that every calorie you eat is of high nutritional quality to help your body resist cravings.

Recent research suggests that up to 30% of obese people suffer from binge eating, a condition associated with eating disorders such as anorexia and bulimia nervosa. Binge eaters are more likely to be depressed and have anxiety disorders, such as panic attacks and post-traumatic stress problems because they keep on using up their available blood sugar and thus need to replenish the supply.

All cases of binge eating, whether associated with obesity or eating disorders, should be treated medically, but there are simple self-help strategies that can alleviate some of the difficulties. Avoiding refined sugar, junk food, caffeine, alcohol, and recreational drugs helps to stabilise blood sugar levels, improve metabolism, and bring greater inner clarity. Eating regular meals containing foods high in calcium, magnesium, zinc, B-vitamins, and vitamin C also helps in this. Getting enough sleep, allowing time for creative expression and spending time outdoors assists in removing internal clutter.

How many calories do we need?

A living body is rather like an internal combustion engine, burning fuel and oxygen to release energy and giving off carbon dioxide and other waste products. This energy is used to maintain healthy functioning of the body and support activity. Not all the energy contained in food is available to the body. This is for two reasons:

1. Not all the food we eat is absorbed through the digestive tract—99% of carbohydrate, 95% of fat, and 92% of protein, in fact.
2. Not all the protein we absorb is converted into energy—some of it is incorporated into the structure of body tissues.

Basal Metabolic Rate (BMR)

Of the energy that is available, a great deal is used to maintain the basal metabolic rate (BMR). This is a measure of the energy needed to fuel all basic life functions while we are at rest. As well as the BMR, physical activity accounts for about 20–40% of our energy use, with digestion, temperature regulation, and coping with the after-effects of physical exertion accounting for the rest.

There are a number of factors that cause variation in energy needs between individuals:

1. Body size—the bigger you are, the more energy you will need to perform the same activities. Energy use is also affected by body composition. A well-muscled body burns more energy than a fat body, which explains why it is easier to keep a fit body trim.
2. Age—babies use a lot of energy to keep warm, and children and teenagers need extra energy to grow and fuel their often vigorous physical activities. As we get older, our metabolism slows down, our body tissues become more fatty, and we tend to become less active. Consequently, we need a lower intake of energy to maintain a healthy weight.
3. Sex—men generally need more calories than women because their body tissues contain less fat, their BMR is higher, and they are on average bigger. Pregnant women need extra energy to support the growth of the baby, and breastfeeding mothers require extra energy for producing milk.
4. Diet—overeating increases the BMR by 5–10%, while dieting reduces it by the same amount. Herein lies the paradox of weight loss: if you eat less to try to lose weight, your BMR drops, which means that your capacity to burn calories also diminishes. In effect, this means that dieting without an increase in physical activity is unlikely to produce sustainable weight loss. Aerobic exercise helps the process of weight reduction in three ways: first, it draws on energy stores while you are doing it, as well as during the following day when your body is recovering and readjusting. Second, exercise encourages the development of muscle, which raises the BMR. This means that you burn more calories at rest as well as when exercising. Third, exercise improves the circulation, enhances the absorption, digestion, and metabolism of food, and helps the body to rid itself of waste products.

5. Activity—it is normal to eat more if you use a lot of energy for physical activity: athletes and heavy-manual workers have increased energy needs to match their energy output.
6. Climate—keeping the right body temperature consumes energy: shivering to keep warm and sweating to keep cool both use up extra calories.
7. Genetic factors—these account for variations in BMR of up to 10% in people of the same age, sex, and body weight.
8. Hormonal state—thyroid over-activity increases energy expenditure, while thyroid under-activity reduces it. In women, the BMR is higher after ovulation. During pregnancy, the BMR falls initially, then increases as body weight increases.
9. Psychological state—anxiety and chronic stress increase energy expenditure.
10. Drugs—stimulants, such as nicotine and caffeine, increase energy expenditure. Amphetamines and other stimulants are sometimes used in treatment of obesity for this reason. Beta-blockers, often used in the treatment of high blood pressure and heart disease, decrease energy expenditure, and can cause weight gain.
11. Disease—fevers, tumours, and the physiological problems caused by severe burns all increase BMR.

Body Mass Index (BMI)

The Body Mass Index provides a simple method of checking whether your weight is right for your height and build:

1. Write down your weight in kilograms (for example, 70).
2. Measure your height in metres (for example, 1.7).
3. Multiply this number by itself (for example, if you are 1.7 m tall, you would multiply $1.7 \times 1.7 = 2.89$).
4. Divide your weight by your height multiplied by itself (in this example, $70/2.89 = 24.22$). This figure is your BMI.

Though simple to calculate, the BMI provides a powerful way of correlating weight to the likelihood of illness. Individuals with a high BMI are more likely to suffer from diabetes, hypertension, and cardiovascular disease, as well as depression, respiratory disease, and ulcers.

The Body Mass Index is interpreted as follows:

BMI

under 20	=	underweight
20–25	=	healthy weight
25–30	=	overweight
30–35	=	obese
over 35	=	seriously obese

Optimum calorie-intake tables grouped according to age and sex

Children and young people (aged 1–18)
Average daily energy need (moderate activity)

AGE	BOYS	GIRLS
1–3 years	1250 kcal	1175 kcal
4–6 years	1700 kcal	1550 kcal
7–10 years	1975 kcal	1750 kcal
11–14 years	2225 kcal	1850 kcal
15–18 years	2750 kcal	2100 kcal

Adults
Average daily energy need (moderate activity)

AGE	MEN	WOMEN
19–59 years	2700 kcal	2050 kcal
60–75 years	2350 kcal	1900 kcal
75+ years	2100 kcal	1800 kcal

Adjustments

- When involved in heavy activity or vigorous exercise, add 500 kcal per day.
- If leading a sedentary lifestyle, subtract 150 kcal per day.
- During pregnancy, add 200 kcal per day during the last 3 months.
- While breastfeeding, add 500–600 kcal per day during the first 6 months. After that, add between 250 and 550 depending on how much of the baby's energy and nutrient needs are supplied by breast-feeding. As soon as weaning begins, the mother's energy needs begin to fall to pre-pregnancy levels.

CHAPTER 7

All about carbohydrates

There are many types of carbohydrates, and most are essential sources of energy in the human diet. Most of the carbohydrate comes from plants, which convert sunlight into carbohydrates in a process called photosynthesis—in other words, they convert solar energy into chemical energy.

The only significant animal sources of carbohydrates in the human diet are lactose from dairy products and fructose from honey.

Carbohydrate digestion begins in the mouth where chewing breaks up the food and mixes it with a digestive enzyme called amylase. Gastric acid in the stomach breaks the food down further, but the main digestion occurs in the small intestine with the help of enzymes secreted by the pancreas.

Absorption is slowed by eating raw foods, starchy foods, and by the presence of protein and fats.

Carbohydrate that escapes digestion in the small intestine is fermented in the large intestine and turned into fatty acids and gas. The fatty acids are absorbed, and so is the gas to a certain extent, but if too much gas is produced, it is expelled as wind. Absorbed gas is excreted through the lungs.

The fermentation of small polysaccharides (such as inulin found in dandelion root, Jerusalem artichoke, chicory, asparagus, artichoke, onion, garlic, and elecampane) is probiotic. Interestingly, the word *inulin* comes from the Latin name for elecampane, *Inula helenum*.

The fermentation process feeds the gut biome and stimulates the growth of bifido-bacteria. It helps to protect the natural bacterial flora of the digestive tract. Feeding the biome with probiotics is always beneficial but overstimulation can cause a lot of wind and be very uncomfortable. Chewing fennel or cardamom seeds can help.

Monosaccharides and disaccharides

Monosaccharides are simple carbohydrates that contain only one carbohydrate molecule. There are two different types of monosaccharide: glucose and fructose, both of which are found in fruits and vegetables.

Glucose provides the fuel for all the body's metabolic activities. It is either absorbed directly from the digestive tract or released from the breakdown of disaccharides and polysaccharides into monosaccharides during digestion.

Simple sugars (monosaccharides and disaccharides) are found within the cell walls of fruits and vegetables, and can also be extracted from sugar cane, sugar beet, maple, corn or honey. They are very easily absorbed into the bloodstream, and the quick energy boost they provide can seem very attractive when you are feeling low. However, an abundance of sugar in the blood is always followed by a corresponding release of insulin, which promotes the transportation of sugar into cells. This in turn causes a drop in blood sugar levels, followed by a renewed feeling of lethargy and a craving for more sugar.

When two monosaccharides combine, they form disaccharides, such as lactose (milk sugar), sucrose (table sugar), maltose (found in malted wheat and barley), and trehalose (found in mushrooms).

Refined sugar is a disaccharide made from sugar cane and sugar beets, leaving molasses as a by-product. It is associated with a range of health problems including tooth decay, obesity, diabetes, Crohn's disease, candida, heart disease, and cancer.

The average Westerner consumes about 30 kg of refined sugar per year, mostly as an added ingredient in processed foods and drinks. "Raw" cane sugar is less refined and contains sucrose plus small quantities of micronutrients. But it is still sugar!

The food sugars that are most important in human nutrition are the monosaccharides—glucose and fructose—and the disaccharides—sucrose and lactose. Some of the physiological effects of sugars are determined at least as much by their physical form as by their chemical structures.

Sugars are classified into three groups for the purpose of deriving dietary reference values (DRVs):

Non-milk extrinsic, milk extrinsic, and intrinsic

Extrinsic (sugars not contained within cell walls in food)	Milk and milk products = *lactose*
	Non-milk = mainly sucrose (table sugar, baked and processed foods, honey)
Intrinsic (sugars contained within the cell walls of fruit and vegetables)	Fructose Glucose Sucrose (within cell walls)

No adverse effects on dental health or health in general can be attributed to intrinsic sugar. However, non-milk extrinsic sugars play a significant role in causing tooth decay. In its natural form, sugar is combined with plant fibre and is diluted with water, and comes "packaged" with important nutrients, including vitamins and minerals; but when extracted, refined, concentrated, and added to foods such as cakes, biscuits, sweets, and soft drinks, sugar becomes the main cause of tooth decay.

It seems likely that a combination of high sugar and high fat intakes predispose towards diabetes. Epidemiological surveys have shown a strong association between sugar and fat intakes. Sugar makes fat more palatable and is frequently combined with it in cakes, biscuits, confectionery, and many processed foods. The two ingredients together provide a concentrated source of calories that contributes to obesity, and many scientists believe that obesity is a key factor in the aetiology of late-onset diabetes.

Opinions are divided on the effect of milk sugar in the diet. In the majority of the world's population, the ability to digest milk sugar (lactose) decreases after the age of five years, and drinking milk thereafter can lead to bloating, cramps, wind, and diarrhoea. Young people with abdominal pains often suffer from lactose intolerance, which can be relieved by excluding dairy from the diet. People of all ages who suffer from allergies, skin problems, inflammations, and autoimmune disorders, can also benefit from giving up dairy.

Polysaccharides

Polysaccharides are made up of chains of monosaccharides and come in two varieties: starch (complex carbohydrate) and non-starch polysaccharide (fibre).

Plants store energy in the form of complex carbohydrate, which is found in large amounts in grains and roots.

Starch is found in the cell walls of whole grains, vegetables, and raw fruits. During digestion, cell walls are broken down to make the carbohydrates accessible for absorption.

Foods rich in complex carbohydrates are good for health for four reasons:

1. They do not expose the teeth to the effects of "free" sugars.
2. They slow the digestive process, producing a feeling of fullness.
3. They help to maintain stable blood sugar levels.
4. Their non-digestible plant cell walls (fibre) provide bulk for the faeces.

Even though complex carbs are made from the same building blocks as simple sugars, they release their sugar molecules at a much slower rate, producing a more measured insulin response and steadier blood sugar and energy levels.

Fibre (non-starch polysaccharide) is found in plant cell walls where it plays a structural role.

Fibre comes in two forms—soluble and insoluble:

Soluble fibre

Including pectins, gums, and mucilages, is easily digested whereas insoluble fibre, including cellulose, hemicellulose, and lignans, passes through the digestive tract undigested. A high intake of foods naturally rich in soluble and insoluble fibre reduces the risk of gallstones, and may also decrease the risk of coronary heart disease by lowering blood cholesterol levels. Soluble fibre also protects the lining of the digestive tract and reduces the risk of blood clot formation.

Good food sources of soluble fibre include:

- Rolled oats
- Whole grains
- Tropical fruit (including mango, papaya, pineapple, banana)
- Psyllium husk and flax seeds
- Cruciferous vegetables (including Brussels sprouts, cabbage, kale, broccoli)
- Pulses (including beans, lentils, peas)
- Avocado
- Roots (including potato, sweet potato, carrot, turnip)
- Dried fruit (including figs, prunes, apricots, dates)
- Citrus fruit (including orange, lemon, mandarin, grapefruit)
- Fruit (including pear, apple, passion fruit)
- Soft fruit (including peach, nectarine, apricot).

Insoluble fibre

Reduces the time it takes for food to pass through the gut by increasing the bulk of faeces and helps to protect against digestive disorders and cancers.

Foods high in fibre also tend to be rich in health-protective micronutrients, such as vitamins, antioxidants, and phytochemicals, and they help to improve the control of blood sugar levels in diabetes.

High fibre diets give an average digestive "transit time" of 24–48 hours, compared with the average Western diet, which gives an average transit time of 72 hours. A long intestinal transit time is a risk factor for diverticulitis and colon cancer.

Bran fibre, in wholemeal bread and some breakfast cereals, can, paradoxically, cause constipation because it absorbs water from the gut. If you eat a lot of bran, it is important to drink at least 1.5 litres of water per day to counter this effect.

Eating an excess of foods with added fibre may also decrease the absorption of drugs, vitamins, minerals, and other nutrients.

Phytate

Some non-starch polysaccharide components, found especially in wheat bran and cereals, contain a substance called phytate, which may bind minerals such as calcium, zinc, and copper in the gut and make them unavailable for absorption. There is no evidence of any resulting long-term adverse effects but care not to overdo fibre intake should be taken by people, such as the elderly, whose diets may be only just adequate in minerals. In those cases, foods, such as whole grains, fruits, and vegetables may be better sources of fibre than added bran.

Good food sources of insoluble fibre include:

- Wheat bran, wheat germ, and oat bran
- Whole grains, pasta, and bread
- Pulses (including beans, lentils, and peas)
- Berries
- Leafy greens
- Dried fruit
- Nuts
- Apples and pears with skin.

Resistant starch

Refers to carbohydrates that escape digestion in the small intestine and reach the large intestine where it is consumed or fermented by colonic bacteria (the gut biome or microbiota). Fermentation of resistant starch produces short-chain fatty acids and increases the bacterial cell mass. The fatty acids are absorbed from the colon.

Resistant starch reduces the glycaemic response to food, and may also reduce appetite, and reduce blood cholesterol levels.

Good food sources of resistant starch include:

- cold cooked potatoes
- cold cooked rice
- chickpeas
- lentils
- cold cooked pasta
- cereals
- red kidney beans
- green peas
- underripe banana
- rolled oats
- brown rice
- Jerusalem artichoke.

Carbohydrate loading

Carbohydrates can be stored in the liver and muscles in the form of glycogen, which, when required, is converted back to glucose for use as a fuel. This process is under the dual control of the hormones insulin and glucagon and allows endurance athletes to continue competing long after blood glucose has been exhausted as a source of fuel. "Carbohydrate loading" is commonly used by endurance athletes before a competition. It involves increasing the intake of unrefined carbohydrate foods—such as grains, wholemeal bread, potatoes, and pasta, for 1–4 days immediately before an event.

Glycaemic index

Developed by Dr David Jenkins and others in Toronto in 1981, the Glycaemic Index (GI) ranks foods according to how quickly they are digested and how quickly the carbohydrates in them are absorbed into the bloodstream from the digestive tract.

The Glycaemic Index ranks carbohydrate-containing foods on as scale from 0 to 100, according to how much they raise your body's blood sugar levels after you have eaten them. The higher the number on the GI scale, the faster your body digests and absorbs the food, resulting in bigger fluctuations in blood sugar levels—the energy highs and lows we experience of the course of a day.

Choosing low-GI carbs causes less fluctuation in blood glucose and insulin levels, which is beneficial in the management of diabetes and the prevention of heart disease, and when you are trying to lose weight sustainably.

For single foods, a low GI value is associated with improved blood sugar control, to keep energy levels balanced, increased insulin sensitivity, and a reduction in fat and cholesterol levels in the bloodstream. Low-GI foods will also help prolong physical endurance, giving you power for longer, which also helps with weight management.

The glycaemic load is the combination of the GI of a food and the amount of carbs it contains in a normal portion. Diets with a high GI or high glycaemic load are associated with increased risk of insulin insensitivity and type 2 diabetes.

Examples of Foods with high GI (>70)

Cakes, cookies, muffins, and rice cakes, rye crispbread, flour, cornflakes, muesli, puffed rice, shredded wheat, millet, rice, ice cream Banana, mango, pawpaw, orange juice, potatoes, sweet potatoes

Examples of Foods with mid-range GI (56–69)

Apple juice, orange, bulgur, bran, baked beans, black-eyed peas, green peas, pinto beans, white pasta

Examples of Foods with low GI (<55)

Pearl barley, apple, dried apricots, underripe banana, pear, rye kernels, milk, yoghurt, butter beans, chickpeas, haricot beans, kidney beans, lentils, soya beans, small seeds, walnuts, most whole grains

The GI of a food will also depend on:

- Ripeness—the riper the fruit, the more sugar it contains, so the GI will be higher.
- Cooking methods—cooking is a kind of ripening process where the cell walls are broken down, so the more cooked, or overcooked, a food is, the easier it is to digest and the more it will increase the GI.
- Processing—whole grain has a lower GI than flour because the grinding breaks down the cell walls and make the carbs more easily accessible. Mashed potatoes and chips have a higher GI than boiled.
- Storage—stored winter roots and tubers have a higher GI than early summer varieties.

Sugar in alcohol

People have been drinking alcohol for over 9000 years, when the first fermented alcoholic drinks are thought to have been made. Alcohol is produced by fermenting glucose with yeast. The source of the glucose determines which alcoholic beverage it becomes—beer is made from fermented grains flavoured with hops (it is the most consumed alcoholic drink in the world!), cider from fruit juice (most commonly apple), wine from grapes. Spirits, such as whisky, vodka, and gin, are made by repeated distillation of fermented alcohol.

According to the WHO, alcohol is now the leading worldwide cause of disease, disability, and mortality.

Drinking alcohol may cause malnutrition, and it can act as a toxin causing pathological changes to the liver, brain, muscles, gut, and other organs and tissues.

On the other hand, in some people, consuming one or two drinks per day may have a beneficial effect in reducing cardiovascular disease according to recent research, although some studies were carried out by the University of Bordeaux…

The most recent reviews suggest that the cardioprotective effect is minimal or negligible, and also outweighed by the overall detrimental effect. It is thought that only women over the age of 55 benefit from the cardioprotective effect.

Women should avoid drinking in the first trimester of pregnancy as it can lead to neurological problems and low birth weight in the baby. Breastfeeding mothers should also avoid alcohol because the milk will contain traces of alcohol, have a different smell, and may affect the baby's nutritional intake and feeding pattern.

The effects of alcohol misuse

Alcohol misuse is common. On average, 50% of chronic alcohol misusers will have one or more health problems. In Europe and America, 15–55% of people admitted to hospital are alcohol abusers. In London, 30% of all acute hospital admissions are alcohol-related.

Over 200 different alcohol-related problems affect alcoholics:

- 80% have a fatty liver, and 10–15% have cirrhosis of the liver.
- 30% have gastrointestinal problems, and all parts of the digestive system, from the mouth to the rectum, can be affected by alcohol misuse.
- 50% have bone marrow changes and/or skeletal damage, such as osteoporosis, fractures, and post-fracture malunion.
- 20–30% have cardiac abnormalities or other cardiovascular problems such as hypertension.
- 80% have skin problems of vascular, fungal, bacterial, or viral origin.

- 40–60% have alcoholic myopathy (muscular weakness).
- 50% of male alcoholics suffer from infertility and sexual dysfunction.
- 10–15% of chronic alcoholics suffer from organic brain disease.
- 50% have nutritional deficiencies caused by poor dietary intake, empty calories, maldigestion and malabsorption, poor liver function, and increased kidney excretion of nutrients.

Nutritional deficiencies are also common among alcohol misusers, who also tend to eat more junk foods and less fresh fruit and vegetables than teetotallers. Alcohol can also interfere with micronutrients such as B1, B2, folate, iron, zinc, and selenium.

Several types of cancer, including mouth, throat, stomach, colon, liver, and breast, are linked to alcohol misuse, and 3.6% of all cancers are attributed to drinking alcohol. The International Agency for Research on Cancer classifies alcohol as a carcinogen. The higher and more prolonged the intake, the higher the risk, but there is no "safe threshold" as tolerance varies greatly. The form of alcohol consumed makes little difference, as it is the amount and the length of time that matters.

Calories in alcoholic drinks

	kcal/100 ml
Alcohol-free beer	7
Lager	29
Special brew	59
Bitter	30
Cider (dry)	36
Wine (dry, red/white)	67
Wine (white, sweet)	94
Sherry (dry)	116
Spirits (40% proof)	222

Source: MAFF. The Composition of Foods.

CHAPTER 8

All about proteins

Between 10 and 15% of the calories we consume each day come from protein. Although it can be used as an energy source, the main purpose of protein is to provide the building blocks necessary for the growth and maintenance of body structures.

The Estimated Average Requirement (EAR) for protein for adults of all ages in the UK is 0.66g/kg/day. The current average intakes in the UK range from 0.7 to 2.72g/kg/day. The tolerable upper limit (TUL) has not been identified for protein but it is thought that 35% of calories as protein can be eaten without adverse effects.

Expert opinion, however, is divided on the matter, especially as excess animal protein may be implicated in increasing the risk of health problems such as osteoporosis, kidney stones, cancer, coronary heart disease, liver, and kidney problems.

Proteins are complex chemicals, which come in many shapes and sizes. All proteins are compounds of carbon, nitrogen, hydrogen, and oxygen organised into amino acid building blocks. Most proteins contain sulphur, and some contain phosphorus.

They all contain amino acids linked together into chains and folded into specific shapes. Protein chains vary in length from two to thousands of amino acids. There are 20 naturally occurring amino acids used by the body, but the number of ways in which they can be arranged is almost infinite, in the same way as an infinite number of words can be made from an alphabet of 26 letters.

It is the specific and unique sequence of these amino acid subunits, or "letters", which gives each protein its characteristic structural and enzymatic properties.

Amino acids are classified into types: essential, semi-essential, and non-essential. The essential amino acids cannot be made by the body in amounts sufficient for health so they must be obtained from the diet. The non-essential are no less important than essential amino acids but they can be synthesised from other amino acids in the body or the diet as long as there is sufficient protein to make them from. If no protein is eaten, 90% of amino acids can be recycled from worn-out proteins before these are excreted from the body.

If one of the essential amino acids is not provided or recycled in adequate amounts, then it is not possible to maintain the right protein synthesis and balance in the body, regardless of the total intake of protein.

The semi-essential amino acids are normally in plentiful supply but under some circumstances, such as trauma or rapid growth, the need may outstrip the body's capacity to synthesise them, in which case they are also needed in the diet.

Essential and non-essential amino acids

Essential	Semi-Essential	Non-Essential
Histidine	Arginine	Alanine
Isoleucine	Asparagine	Aspartate
Leucine	Cysteine	Glutamate
Lysine	Glutamine	
Methionine	Glycine	
Phenylalanine	Proline	
Threonine	Serine	
Tryptophan	Tyrosine	
Valine		

The quality of animal and plant protein

Earlier recommendations for human protein intake differentiated between "first class" animal protein and "second class" plant protein on the basis that animal proteins had an amino acid content similar to human proteins.

But when the biological value of plant-based proteins is compared to animal-based proteins, it becomes clear that all plant-based proteins contain ALL essential amino acids. Most plant-based proteins contain more essential amino acids than needed, and some plant-based proteins—for example from potatoes—are indistinguishable from animal-based proteins in terms of total amount and balance of essential amino acids. The essential amino acid content in potatoes exceeds the requirement for every one of them, and as potatoes contain 11% of their energy as protein, it is not surprising that they have been the major source of protein in many traditional diets.

The Danish doctor and food scientist Mikkel Hindhede performed many experiments in the early part of the twentieth century to find the minimum requirement for protein. He attempted to starve his subjects of protein by putting them on a diet consisting almost entirely of potatoes, and wanted to see how long it would take before they displayed symptoms of protein deficiency. To his astonishment, his subjects instead became healthier and stronger, even after a year on the potato diet! This led Hindhede to travel to Ireland and America to study populations that based their diet almost entirely on potatoes or other plant-based protein, and he concluded that meat is unnecessary as a source of protein. It is good to see that, a hundred years later, his observations have been proven biochemically.

All green leafy vegetables contain high-quality protein, a fact that has been largely ignored because of their low calorie content, but in some countries, such as Greece, where large amounts of green leaves are traditionally included in the diet, they can be more than adequate as a protein source—as is proven by grazing animals all over the world.

The important findings are that all plants contain all essential amino acids. Legumes and cereals, roots and tubers are the traditional plant-based sources, but as long as you cover your energy need with different plant-based foods, it is very hard to avoid getting enough protein.

It is therefore becoming clear that eating animal-based protein is a choice not based on nutritional need but on taste and tradition.

Getting enough protein

How much protein we need is a difficult question to answer! Human breast milk only contains around 5% of its calories (energy) as protein, and this obviously meets the requirements of the baby. This is partly because babies and growing children use a huge amount of energy, and as we grow older and less active, the ratio between protein and energy requirement changes, and protein deficiency is more likely in the elderly than in children. Protein-dense foods are more important for adults than for babies and children, and protein deficiency is less likely at any age as physical activity increases because the need for calories also increases.

In the past, protein requirements have been set as grams per kilogram of body weight, but it is now becoming clear that energy expenditure is just as important as body size. It is therefore more useful to set the protein requirement as a percentage of calorie intake.

The average requirement for all ages is 0.7 grams of protein per kilo body weight per day. For a person weighing 60 kg, that would be 42 grams of protein per day, or 168 kcal as protein (since 1 gram of protein contains 4 kcal).

If the average energy need for adults is around 2300 kcal, the percentage needed as protein would be 168 / 2300 x 100 = 7%.

Of course, this is only an average, and there is wide variation depending on age, sex, size, and activity level, but it is safe to say that the need must be somewhere between 4 and 15% of total calories.

Percentage of calories from protein in some common foods

Remember that calories are made of carbs, fats, or protein.

If a food isn't very sweet or fatty, it must contain a relatively high percentage of protein.

Food		Energy (kcal) in 100g	Protein (grams)	% of energy
Fruit	Orange	37	1.1	12
	Blackberries	25	0.9	14
	Raspberries	25	1.4	22
	Strawberries	27	0.8	12
	Blueberries	30	0.6	8
	Apricot, dried	132	3.4	10
Nuts	Almonds	612	21.2	14
	Peanuts	564	25.6	18
	Pumpkin seeds	570	24.4	17
	Sesame seeds	598	18.2	12
	Sunflower seeds	582	19.8	14
Roots	Beetroot	36	1.7	19
	Potato	72	1.8	10
Pulses	Baked beans	81	4.8	24
	Chickpeas	121	8.4	28
	Green beans	24	1.9	32
	Lentils	105	8.8	34
	Green peas	83	6.9	33
	Soya beans	141	14	40
Grains	Oats	401	12.4	12
	Quinoa	309	13.8	18
	Rice	141	2.6	7
	Wheat	310	12.7	16
Vegetables	Artichoke hearts	18	2.8	62
	Asparagus	31	3.6	46
	Broccoli	34	4.2	49
	Cauliflower	34	3.6	42
	Curly kale	33	3.4	41
	Lettuce	10	0.7	30
	Mushrooms	13	1.8	55
	Spinach	25	2.8	45

(Continued)

(Continued)

Food		Energy (kcal) in 100g	Protein (grams)	% of energy
Meat	Beef steak	246	14.6	47
	Lamb chop	244	15.2	25
	Bacon	477	24.1	20
	Chicken	259	27.1	42
Fish	Lemon sole, steamed	109	24.7	91
	Salmon, grilled	215	24.2	45
	Tuna, canned	99	23.5	95
	Prawns, boiled	98	23	91
Milk	Whole cow's milk	66	3.3	20
	Soya milk, unsweetened	26	2.4	37
Eggs	Chicken eggs, boiled	148	12.6	34

Source: MAFF. The Composition of Foods.

Protein digestion

Proteins are digested in the stomach and the small intestine where they are absorbed as amino acids. A small amount of proteins is also absorbed whole and broken down into amino acids by the liver, where all amino acids are processed before they are distributed in the bloodstream to become part of enzymes, body cells, hormones, hair, nails, bones, muscles, and DNA.

The body is continually combining and recombining amino acids to make new proteins, and nearly all body cells are capable of synthesising specific proteins for their own purposes. Worn-out proteins are dismantled by the liver and excreted in the urine via the kidneys, as is any excess protein.

The body maintains a protein reserve of between three and four hundred grams to compensate for variations in protein requirement and intake.

The absorption of carbohydrate into the bloodstream stimulates the release of insulin from the pancreas. In addition to promoting the uptake of glucose into body cells, insulin encourages protein synthesis in the muscles and liver, and inhibits protein breakdown. As long as there are calories available from carbohydrate, there is no need to use body protein for energy and, unlike fat and carbohydrate, protein is used as a source of energy only under exceptional circumstances such as starvation, serious injury, or major disease, such as cancer.

During fasting and in times of trauma or stress, another hormone, called glucagon, is released from the pancreas. Glucagon encourages the body to use amino acids instead of carbohydrates for fuel. The stress hormones cortisol and adrenalin act in a similar way, causing protein in muscles to be broken down into free amino acids for conversion into energy. Trauma and stress can therefore cause the loss of substantial amounts of protein, especially from muscle tissue.

The reason for this may be that the brain normally consumes over half of our daily carbohydrate requirement, especially as glucose, and it requires over 10% more energy when we are exposed to stress. If the hypothalamus registers that the brain lacks glucose, it blocks information from the rest of the body and the stress hormones divert the body's energy consumption to burning protein.

Protein absorption and processing

Deficient secretion of protein-splitting enzymes by the glands of the alimentary tract can affect protein absorption just as much as variation in protein intake. The method of cooking is also very important. Overheating, especially in the absence of water (as in frying) can destroy or inactivate some amino acids, especially lysine.

The standard view is that proteins are broken down into component amino acids during digestion. It is also generally accepted that this breakdown is necessary to allow proteins to be absorbed through the intestinal wall, since they are too large to pass through it in any other way. However, whole proteins can be ingested by lymphocytes lying close to the intestinal lumen in organised lymphoid nodules—Peyer's patches, for example—and carried via the portal circulation to the liver. Such protein is antigenic, and is thus likely to be engulfed by the liver macrophages or passed to macrophages in the tissues. The immunological implications are clearly important, but nutritional significance was added when it became apparent from radioactive tracer studies that whole proteins can also pass through *ordinary* intestinal cells by pinocytosis, and that this route forms a proportion of all protein absorption.

Such findings suggest that need for a complete re-evaluation of protein metabolism to bring the sciences of immunology and nutrition closer together.

The proteins in food, such as casein, lactoglobulins, lactalbumins, and gluten, are triggering agents of food allergy, and so the knowledge that *whole* proteins are potentially able to find their way from the diet to all tissues of the body is obviously significant and may explain a number of allergic syndromes such as migraine, cluster headaches, catarrh, asthma, and gastrointestinal disturbances like irritable bowel.

High-protein diets

Although high-protein paleo diets are popular among weight watchers and body builders, there is doubt in the scientific community about the wisdom of recommending high protein intakes above the recommended daily allowance for adults. But there is currently no reasonable scientific basis for advocating protein consumption above the recommended daily allowance for healthy adults due to the potential health risks involved.

The potential adverse effects of a high-protein supplements and of long-term high meat intake include osteoporosis, liver problems, kidney problems and stones, gout and other inflammatory conditions, cancer, coronary heart disease, and stroke.

The high-protein diets promoted for muscle development, performance-enhancement, and fat loss could be harmful for healthy individuals because the extra protein not used by the body may pose a metabolic burden on bones, kidneys, and liver. The excess protein may also be associated with cardiovascular problems because of the higher intake of saturated fat and cholesterol. The increased intake of purines, which are precursors of uric acid, which in turn can cause gout and kidney stones, and the high intake of sulphur-containing amino acids also increase urinary acidity, which may lead to calcium release from bones and excretion via the kidneys and calcium kidney stone formation.

Gluten

Gluten is the name given to proteins found in wheat, rye, and barley. It makes up 75–85% of the total protein in bread wheat. It is popular because it adds elasticity to flour, like a glue, and it helps foods maintain their shape and give them a chewy texture.

Watch out for gluten in breads, baked goods, pasta, cereals, soups, sauces, dressings, beer, brewer's yeast, food colouring, and malt. It is also a common additive, so read labels, if you want to avoid it.

Oats is gluten-free but is often grown, stored, and milled next to the gluten-containing grains. Eat only oats labelled gluten-free if you wish to avoid gluten in your diet. Maize and rice are gluten-free.

The problem with gluten is that it can trigger allergy, sensitivity and inflammation. "Gluten-related disorders" is an umbrella term for diseases triggered by gluten. These include coeliac disease, non-coeliac gluten sensitivity, wheat allergy, gluten ataxia, and dermatitis herpetiformis.

Coeliac disease affects 1–2% of the population but is often undiagnosed and untreated because the symptoms can be diffuse and difficult to recognise. Untreated coeliac disease may cause malabsorption, iron deficiency, osteoporosis, and general malaise. It is also associated with autoimmune disease such as diabetes, thyroid problems, and skin problems such as dermatitis and psoriasis.

The treatment of coeliac disease requires lifelong exclusion of gluten from the diet. The British Society of Gastroenterology and Coeliac UK also recommends all coeliac disease sufferers consume 1000 mg of calcium per day.

CHAPTER 9

All about fats

Fats are energy-dense foods containing 9 kcal per gram—more than twice as much as carbohydrate or protein. They supply the body with essential fatty acids, carry fat-soluble vitamins, aid metabolism, and provide structure for cell membranes. They also make food taste good.

Body fat is our energy store which we draw on whenever our diet is lacking in calories. Excess fat and carbohydrate in the diet increases the amount of body fat, while fasting causes fat breakdown. Many drugs and toxins find their way into fatty tissues, so fasting is a powerful way to detox the body.

Fats contain fatty acids, which are long hydrocarbon chains with a carboxyl group attached to one end. There are three main types of fatty acids, classified according to the organisation of the hydrogen atoms in their chains—saturated, monounsaturated, and polyunsaturated. About 16 different fatty acids make up the bulk of the fatty acids in food.

Saturated fatty acids (SFA)

A saturated fatty acid contains the maximum possible number of hydrogen atoms, so they have no double bonds in their chemical structure. This makes them very stable. The most abundant saturated fatty acids in foods are myristic acid with 14 carbon atoms in the chain (C14), palmitic acid with 16 carbon atoms (C16), and stearic acid (C18).

Myristic acid gets its name from nutmeg, *Myristica fragrans*, which contains about 75% myristic acid; it is also found in coconut oil, palm kernel oil, and butter.

Palmitic acid is the most common saturated fatty acid found in animals, plants, and microorganisms, but it was first discovered in palm oil, hence the name. It is also present in breast milk, dairy fat, meat, cocoa butter, and as an additive to many processed foods.

Stearic acid is a waxy solid named after the Greek word for tallow and, except for palmitic acid, is the most common saturated fatty acid found in nature. It is most abundant in animal fat, shea butter, and cocoa butter, and as a food additive (E570).

Saturated fatty acids are usually solid at room temperature. They can be made in the body so are not essential in the diet.

Monounsaturated fatty acids (MUFA)

A monounsaturated fatty acid is usually a long chain of fatty acids in which two hydrogen atoms are missing, so they have one double bond in their chemical structure. Because they have room for two extra hydrogen atoms, they are less solid than saturated fats, and they exist as thick oils at room temperature.

The most common monounsaturated fatty acid in nature is oleic acid (C18), named after olive oil, which contains 70% oleic acid. It is also found in avocado, nuts, palm oil, and some animal fats and fatty fish. Monounsaturated oil is thought to protect against heart disease by lowering blood cholesterol levels. It can be made by the body so is not essential in the diet.

Monounsaturated oil is the best choice for cooking because MUFA react less to heat than saturated or polyunsaturated oils.

Polyunsaturated fatty acids (PUFA)

A polyunsaturated fatty acid is usually a long-chain fatty acid in which more than two hydrogen atoms are missing, so they have two to six double bonds. The most common ones are linoleic acid with four hydrogen atoms missing, and linolenic acid with six hydrogen atoms missing. These two polyunsaturated fatty acids are known as the essential fatty acids (EFA) because they cannot be made by the body and are therefore essential in the diet.

Linoleic acid is an omega-6 fatty acid. Linolenic acid exists in two forms: gamma-linolenic acid, which is an omega-6 fatty acid, and alpha-linolenic acid, which is an omega-3 fatty acid.

Humans have a specific requirement for linoleic acid and alpha-linolenic acid. Although deficiency does not occur in people eating a "normal" diet, it is estimated that linoleic acid should provide at least 1% and alpha-linolenic acid at least 0.2% of total energy intake.

Both linoleic and linolenic acid can be converted in the body to long-chain polyunsaturated fatty acids, which are important components of cell membranes.

In the brain, essential fatty acids and their derivatives are the major components of membrane phosphoglycerides, especially in the synaptic membranes. In the foetus and newborn baby, 70% of all essential fatty acid intake goes to the brain. The demand for essential fatty acids increases wherever tissue growth is taking place. The daily requirements are also much increased during illness and convalescence.

A second major function of PUFAs is in the biosynthesis of prostaglandins and the control of platelet function. A meal containing appreciable amounts of saturated fatty acids will decrease blood clotting time, that is increase the tendency for clots to form, whereas a similar meal, but high in polyunsaturated fatty acids, will not change clotting time.

Omega-6 fatty acids are found in most vegetables oils and are thought to lower blood cholesterol and low-density lipoproteins (LDLs). Oily fish, soya beans, evening primrose oil, walnuts, flax seeds, and pumpkin seeds are rich in omega-3 fatty acids, which reduce inflammation and protect the heart.

Polyunsaturated fatty acids are found in abundance in vegetable oils such as sunflower, soyabean, safflower seed, and corn. They are the thinnest oils, liquid even at cool temperatures, and are sensitive to heat, light, and air; they tend to go rancid unless kept in a cool, dark place.

Whether there is an upper safe limit for polyunsaturated fatty acid consumption is not known, but diets containing as much as 15% of the total dietary energy as linoleic acid seem to have no adverse effect.

Fatty acid composition of some fats and oils (fatty acids per cent of total fatty acids)

Vegetable	% SFA	% MUFA	% PUFA
Coconut	90	7	3
Corn	17	31	52
Olive	15	73	12
Palm	47	44	9
Peanut, groundnut, arachis	20	50	30
Rapeseed	6	67	26
Safflower	11	13	76
Soya bean	15	25	60
Sunflower	14	33	52
Vegetable margarine, soft	33	44	23
Vegetable margarine, hard	38	49	13
Animal			
Butter	66	26	3
Compound cooking fat	42	42	15
Lard	44	44	10
Suet	58	37	2
Low fat spread	28	40	31
Margarine, mixed oils, hard	38	45	16
Margarine, mixed oils, soft	31	47	20

Source: MAFF. The Composition of Foods.

Trans fats

Unsaturated fats are sometimes turned into saturated trans fats by a chemical process called hydrogenation. This happens naturally in some animal fats, such as beef and milk fat, owing to hydrogenation of polyunsaturated fatty acids in the rumen of the animal. (The rumen is the largest stomach compartment in ruminant animals, which are hoofed herbivorous grazing animals, including cows and sheep, with specialised stomachs that can ferment plant-based foods into a so-called "cud", which is regurgitated and chewed at leisure, a process known as rumination.)

The total trans fat content in beef, milk, butter, cheese, curds and tallow it is 5–10%. Trans fatty acids are also sometimes found in processed foods and vegetable margarines when unsaturated fats are hydrogenated saturated fats because of their higher melting point for use in foods such as margarines. This is the reason some of the figures in the table above do not all add up to 100%.

But health concerns have been raised over excessive intake of trans fats, and they have been linked to a number of health problems, including cancer, atherosclerosis, and infertility. For this reason, manufacturers now normally use other methods of preparing fats that do not form trans fats. To avoid trans fats, limit the amount of animal fats you eat and choose products marked "no trans fats" or "unhydrogenated" whenever possible.

Cholesterol and lipoproteins

Cholesterol and steroid hormones are made from sterols. High levels of cholesterol in the blood increase the risk of cardiovascular disease. Despite its bad reputation, cholesterol is a vital component of cell membranes, and it is involved in the production of bile acids and sex hormones. It is not necessary to eat cholesterol, however, because the body makes all that it needs.

Meat, shellfish, eggs, and dairy products tend to have a high cholesterol content, and foods rich in cholesterol also tend to have a high content of saturated fat.

Lipoprotcins are particles in the circulation with the task of "shuttling" cholesterol and fat molecules (lipids) to tissues where they are needed. Lipoproteins have traditionally been classified in four main groups according to their density: chylomicrons, very-low-lipoproteins (VLDLs), low-density lipoproteins (LDLs), and high-density lipoproteins (HDLs). Recently, a fifth category has been added, a type of LDL called lipoprotein (a) (LPa) because it has been found to have a strong independent association with the formation of atherosclerosis.

All the LDLs are the main carriers of cholesterol in the blood, and they are known as "bad" lipoproteins because they are associated with high blood cholesterol levels and can form blockages called plaques, also known as atherosclerosis or hardening of the arteries. LPas are stickier than other types of LDLs, and they are more likely to cause blockages and blood clots in the arteries, increasing the risk of coronary heart disease and stroke.

High-density lipoproteins (HDLs) are known as "good" lipoproteins because they mop up excess cholesterol and return it to the liver for reprocessing and excretion. HDLs also remove cholesterol from clogged-up arteries, helping to prevent cardiovascular disease.

To reduce the level of LDLs, it is helpful to avoid meat and dairy products in your diet; losing weight, not smoking, reducing stress, getting regular exercise, and lowering your blood pressure are also beneficial. More than 50% of UK adults have elevated total and LDL cholesterol levels.

Foods that are known to lower blood cholesterol levels include:

- Oats
- Barley and other whole grains
- Beans
- Aubergine
- Okra
- Nuts and seeds
- Vegetable oils
- Fruit, particularly apples, grapes, strawberries, and citrus fruits, because they are rich in the soluble fibre 'pectin' that lowers LDLs
- Foods, herbs, and supplements containing sterols and stanols; 2 grams per day can lower LDL cholesterol by 10%
- Soya: edamame beans, tofu, tempeh, soya milk
- Psyllium seeds.

All of the above lower blood cholesterol levels by delivering soluble fibre, which binds cholesterol so it can be excreted from the body, or by providing HDL polyunsaturated fats, which directly lower LDLs, or by containing plant sterols and stanols, which block cholesterol absorption.

The cholesterol content of some common foods

Food	Cholesterol content mg per 100g
Plant-based foods (all grains, nuts, fruits, vegs, etc.)	0
Dairy products	
Cow's milk	14
Human milk	16
Butter	230
Cream	140
Cheese, average	100
Eggs	450
Yoghurt	7
Fats and oils	
Animal fats, average	70
Vegetable oils	0
Meat	
Bacon	87
Beef	82
Chicken	97
Lamb	110
Pork	110
Offal	
Brain/brawn (lamb, calf)	2650
Heart (sheep, ox)	245
Kidney (lamb, ox, pig)	667
Liver (calf, lamb, ox, pig)	333
Fish	
White fish, average	70
Fatty fish, average	80
Shellfish	
Lobster	150
Prawns and shrimps	200
Mussels	100
Oysters	50

Source: MAFF. The Composition of Foods.

Dietary fat guidelines (as a percentage of total daily energy intake)

Fat type	Recommended daily intake	Current population daily intake
Total fat	30% or less	35.3%
SFA	10% or less	13.3%
MUFA	12%	13%
PUFA	6%—maximum 10%	6%
Trans fats	Less than 2%	0.5%
Cholesterol	Less than 300 mg	Not known

Fat guidelines

- Keep your daily fat intake at or below 30% of your total calorie intake.
- Keep the ratio of unsaturated to saturated fat in your diet to at least 2:1—that is to say, eat twice as many foods containing unsaturated fats as those containing saturated fats.
- Include omega-3 fatty acids in your diet by eating walnuts and flax seed, or by taking drops of evening primrose or borage oil.
- Eat more low-fat protein foods, such as pulses and green leaves, and reduce the amount of red meat, offal, eggs, and dairy products you eat.
- Avoid foods that are high in cholesterol, such as meat, dairy, and eggs, or keep them to a minimum in your diet.

Fats in food

Fat is the second most important source of energy in the diet, and it accounts for up to 50% of total energy intake in humans. It provides a more concentrated source of energy than carbohydrate or protein, yielding 9 kcal per gram.

Fat is necessary in the diet to allow the absorption of the fat-soluble vitamins.

Fat can be divided into two types: visible fats, such as oil, butter and margarine, and invisible fats, such as the fat in nuts, seeds, beans, fish, meat, and dairy.

Most foods contain at least some fat. Oily fish, vegetable oils, nuts, seeds, olives, avocados, meats, dairy products, and table fats are all examples of high-fat foods, but the types of fatty acids they contain vary.

Olive oil is the best-known source of monounsaturated fat. Vegetable foods contain mostly polyunsaturated fat and, together with oily fish, are the main sources of essential fatty acids in the diet.

Virtually all of the fat in lean white fish is found in the liver, whereas oily fish carry their fat reserves in their flesh.

Meat and dairy products contain mostly saturated fats. However, the composition of the fat depends on the animal's diet and lifestyle. Active animals, fed on pasture and grains, have lower saturated fat content in their meat than those reared using intensive farming methods.

Oils sold as "edible vegetable oils" generally contain a mixture of soya bean and rape seed oils. Rape seed oil contains a long-chain mono-unsaturated fatty acid called erucic acid, which has been shown in animal experiments to cause heart muscle degeneration in rats. There is no evidence that erucic acid does the same thing in humans. However, food manufacturers are compelled by law to limit the amount of erucic acid in edible vegetable oils to below 5% of the total.

Fat absorption and digestion

After eating a meal containing a high proportion of fat, food stays in the stomach for longer than it would after a low-fat meal. This is because fat has to be emulsified by bile in the small intestine before it can be digested. The emulsified fat is broken down by lipases secreted from the pancreas into fatty acids and then absorbed in the small intestine. After absorption, much of the fat is carried as "chylomicrons" in the lymphatic system and then released into the bloodstream via the thoracic duct. Chylomicrons are globules of fat surrounded by a shell of protein. If the production of bile or lipases is impaired then fats are poorly absorbed and the faeces become light or white—as for example in hepatitis, pancreatitis, and obstructive jaundice.

Over 50% of the energy in breast milk comes from fat. This concentrated supply of energy helps support rapid growth. On the other hand, high fat intake (>40% of energy intake) in adults is associated with several diseases of affluence, notably coronary heart disease, obesity, and cancer of the large intestine. For this reason, high fat intakes are considered undesirable for adults. However, at least 10% of energy intake should come from fats to enable the absorption of the oil-soluble vitamins. An ideal level of fat in the diet of adults is probably somewhere between 10 and 30% of the energy intake.

Fat and disease

The Royal College of Physicians advocates a generous intake of polyunsaturated fatty acids but a restricted intake of saturated fatty acids for the prevention of coronary heart disease. High levels of blood fats, especially cholesterol, are associated with an increased risk of coronary heart disease. Blood cholesterol levels are mainly determined by the amount of saturated and polyunsaturated fatty acids in the diet and to a lesser extent by dietary cholesterol. Saturated fatty acids raise blood cholesterol levels; polyunsaturated fatty acids have a cholesterol-lowering effect.

More than 20 studies in 14 different countries have shown that, along with high blood pressure, smoking, and social class, plasma levels of cholesterol and LDL-fats are key factors associated with heart disease.

There is also evidence from different countries that as dietary intake of linoleic acid increases, deaths from coronary heart disease decrease.

Evidence also suggests that PUFAs known as long-chain omega-3 fatty acids, such as eicosapentaeonoic (EPA) and docosahexaenoic acids (from fish oils) have beneficial effects on blood fat levels and may inhibit thrombosis. There is apparently no EPA or docosahexaenoic acids in plant-based diets, but another omega-3 fatty acid, linolenic acid, is present in plants (especially in walnuts, flax seed oil, wheat germ oil, rape seed oil, soya beans, tofu, and seaweed). Linolenic acid can be converted in the body to EPA.

In the UK in 2022, 68% of men and 60% of women were overweight (BMI >25), and 29% of men and 27% of women were considered obese (BMI >30). This means that more than 6 in 10 adults in the UK are overweight or obese, a problem that is associated with deprivation.

Overweight and obesity are the UKs biggest cause of cancer after smoking. Being overweight has many negative effects on the body, including heart problems, diabetes, muscle and bone problems, and increased cancer risk. Obesity is also linked with cardiovascular disease, high blood pressure, diabetes, mental health problems, and certain cancers, including cancers of the womb, breast, kidney, bowel, liver, and gallbladder. A high-fat diet is also linked to the development of late-onset diabetes.

Fatty foods and empty calories contribute particularly to the problem of obesity because of their high calorie and low nutrient content.

Increased access to fresh fruits, vegetables, and unprocessed plant-based foods, as well as awareness of their importance for health and wellbeing could solve this problem for a large part of the population.

Lowering cholesterol

You can reduce cholesterol levels simply by changing what you eat. Cholesterol is only found in animal fats, so if you, for example, are a fan of cheeseburgers, eating less meat (and leaner cuts) and more vegetables, fruits, and whole grains can lower your total cholesterol intake by 25% or more. Cutting back on saturated fat (found in meat and dairy products) and trans fat (partially hydrogenated oils) can reduce cholesterol by 5% to 10%.

Risk factors you can treat or control

You can take steps to address these risk factors:

- hypertension (blood pressure at or above 140/90 mm Hg)
- high levels of triglycerides, LDL cholesterol, or both
- metabolic syndrome, a cluster of cardiovascular risk factors
- overweight (BMI of 25 or more).

Risk factors you can modify or change

You can adjust your lifestyle to minimise or eliminate these risk factors:

- smoking
- physical inactivity
- a diet high in saturated and trans fats
- chronic stress
- social isolation, anxiety, and depression.

Lifestyle research

Lifestyle research shows that:

- Lowering your total blood cholesterol by 10% can decrease your heart attack risk considerably (by 20% to 30%).
- Walking at least two hours a week can cut your chances of dying early from cardiovascular disease by up to 53%.
- If you quit smoking, your risk for heart attack drops by half within a year.
- Maintaining a healthy body weight cuts your risk for heart disease by 45%.
- Eating about 3 grams less salt a day can reduce the need for hypertension treatment by half. It can also decrease deaths from stroke by 22% and those from heart disease by 16%. The easiest way to reduce salt intake is to stop eating convenience foods and meat.

Choosing a cholesterol-lowering diet

If you change your diet away from meat, dairy, and convenience foods to one that is low in saturated fat and made up mostly of fruits, vegetables, and whole grains, you can potentially reduce the risk of heart attack or stroke by 73%.

Foods with the highest cholesterol content, mg per 100g

Brain/brawn (lamb, calf)	2650
Kidney (lamb, ox pig)	667
Eggs	450
Liver (calf, lamb, ox, pig)	333
Heart (sheep, ox)	245
Butter	230
Prawns and shrimps	200
Lobster	150
Cream	140
Lamb, pork	110
Mussels	100
Cheese, average	100

(Continued)

Foods with the highest cholesterol content, mg per 100g (Continued)	
Chicken	97
Bacon	87
Beef	82
Fatty fish, average	80
White fish, average	70
Plant-based foods (all nuts, grains, fruit, vegs, etc.)	0

Healthy eating isn't easy with so much temptation around, but it can be done with a few adjustments, for example:

- Nuts, seeds, and dried fruit instead of cheese and crackers
- Apples, bananas, and oranges instead of muffins or ice cream
- Smoothies or fizzy water with juice or cordial instead of sugar-sweetened drinks.

The health benefits gained by such changes make them well worth the effort.

Four steps for using your diet to lower your cholesterol

1. **Stick with unsaturated fats and avoid saturated and trans fats.** Most vegetable fats (oils) are made up of unsaturated fats that are healthy for your heart. Foods that contain healthy fats include oily fish, nuts, seeds, and vegetables such as avocado. At the same time, limit your intake of foods high in saturated fat, which is found in meat and dairy products, and stay away from trans fats (hardened unsaturated fatty acids found in manufactured meats, including butter and any foods made with "partially hydrogenated vegetable oils"). Avoid red meat, eggs, cow's milk, and cheese, and a decrease in overall fat intake by avoiding table fats (such as butter). Foods containing invisible fat (such as mayonnaise, cakes and rich sauces, and soups) can also make a major contribution to lowering blood cholesterol levels.
2. **Get more soluble fibre.** Eat more soluble fibre, such as that found in oats, linseed, and fresh fruits and vegetables. This type of fibre can significantly lower blood cholesterol level when eaten as part of a healthy-fat diet.
3. **Include plant sterols and stanols in your diet.** These naturally occurring compounds are similar in structure to cholesterol. When

you eat them, they help limit the amount of cholesterol your body can absorb. Plant sterols and stanols are found in an increasing number of food products such as spreads, juices, and soya yoghurt.

4. **Find the diet that works for you.** There is no one-size-fits-all diet for cholesterol control. You may need to try several approaches to find one that works for you. Although diet can be a simple and powerful way to improve cholesterol levels, it plays a bigger role for some people than for others. If your doctor suggests a lower-fat, lower-cholesterol diet, and despite your best efforts it isn't working, you may need a different kind of diet, or medication, or both to bring cholesterol down. Make a gradual change away from processed and convenience foods, and exchanging them for fresh fruits, vegetables, nuts, seeds, pulses and whole grain foods reduces blood-cholesterol levels.

Cholesterol-lowering medicinal herbs and foods

Foods that are known to lower blood cholesterol levels include:

- Oats, psyllium seeds, and linseeds
- Alfalfa sprouts
- Barley and other whole grains
- Beans
- Aubergine
- Okra
- Nuts and seeds
- Vegetable oils
- Globe artichoke: enhances liver function and helps regulate blood fat levels
- Fruit, particularly apples, grapes, strawberries, and citrus fruits, because they are rich in the soluble fibre 'pectin', which lowers LDL
- Foods, herbs, and supplements containing sterols and stanols. (2 grams per day can lower LDL cholesterol by 10%.)
- Soya: edamame beans, tofu, tempeh, soya milk. Recent research recommends that adults should aim to consume 25 g of soya protein daily to lower cholesterol.

Ginger stimulates digestion and peripheral circulation. It also helps lower blood pressure and cholesterol levels.

Garlic is an excellent blood cleanser and thinner and, if used regularly, is efficient in keeping blood-cholesterol levels under control. It can also be good blood pressure-lowering remedy.

Carnitine is a vitamin-like compound, made from the amino acid lysine (with the help of iron and vitamin C), which increases the metabolism of saturated fats and cholesterol. Good sources include tempeh, lentils, muesli, green peas, tahini, chickpeas, beans, nuts and seeds.

Avocado acts as a mild vasodilator, relaxing the muscles surrounding blood vessels and thus reducing blood pressure. Some 80% of the fat in avocado is oleic acid, which reduces blood cholesterol. It also contains beta-sitosterols, which reduce the absorption of cholesterol from food. (Beta-sitosterols are widely used in the manufacture of blood-cholesterol-lowering drugs.)

Niacin (vitamin B3) helps normalise blood pressure and cholesterol. Good sources are breakfast cereals, almonds, wheat germ, tempeh, and oyster mushrooms.

Chlorophyll (green plant pigment) is known for its cholesterol-lowering effect. Good sources include dark leafy greens (spinach, kale, chard, parsley), grasses (wheat, barley, alfalfa), sea vegetables (nori, wakame, kombu) and algae (chlorella, spirulina, blue–green algae).

Specific herbs: milk thistle, dandelion root, lime flowers, fenugreek. Hawthorn berries and flowering tops strengthen the heart muscle and lower blood pressure and blood-cholesterol levels.

CHAPTER 10

All about vitamins

Vitamins are a group of micronutrients that are needed for normal cell function, growth, and development.

There are 13 essential vitamins required for the body to work well. They are divided into two main categories: the fat-soluble A, D, E, and K—found mainly in fatty foods; and those soluble in water—the B-group and vitamin C.

Vitamins are essential nutrients required in small amounts in the diet. The majority cannot be made by the body. However, vitamin D is synthesised in the skin and hair of humans and animals, and in fungi, moss, and algae in response to daylight; vitamin B3 (niacin) is synthesised from tryptophan (an essential amino acid), and vitamin B12 and K are synthesised by bacteria in the intestines and the soil.

The fat-soluble vitamins (A, D, E, K), and vitamin A are poorly soluble in water, so they are chaperoned by transporter proteins and lipoproteins in the circulation.

Classification of vitamins

Fat-soluble vitamins		
A		Retinol
Pro-vitamin A		Beta-carotene
		Carotenoids
D	D2	Ergocalciferol
	D3	Cholecalciferol
E		Tocopherols
K		Phylloquinone
		Menaquinone

Water-soluble vitamins		
B-group:	B1	Thiamin
	B2	Riboflavin
	B3	Niacin
	B5	Pantothenic acid
	B6	Pyridoxine
	B7	Biotin
	B9	Folate and folic acid
	B12	Cobalamin
C		Ascorbic acid

Vitamins are absorbed in the small intestine, especially the fat-soluble vitamins, so people who have had part of their small intestine surgically removed can develop fat-soluble vitamin deficiency.

The large intestine (the colon) is the absorption site for most of the water-soluble vitamins because they are synthesised there by the microbiome. This is one reason why having a healthy microbiome is so important. Diet, drugs, obesity, and diabetes all affect the microbiome. Fermented foods and prebiotics contain naturally synthesised vitamins and increase their production and absorption.

Fresh fruit and vegetables contain more vitamins than other classes of food. Vitamin content is lowered when food is cooked or dried. Lemons, oranges, and other citrus fruits retain their vitamin content even when cooked. Milk is rich in vitamins, which are partially destroyed by pasteurisation and sterilisation. Cow's milk contains more vitamins in summer than in winter and more when the cows are kept on good pasture than when fed formula foods such as in intensive farming systems where animals are kept indoors all year.

Potatoes, carrots, and other root vegetables are rich in vitamin B and C, and particularly retain them after cooking. Scurvy, which at one time was almost universal in Europe, virtually disappeared after the introduction of potatoes from America.

In cereals, the vitamins and mineral salts are contained chiefly in the outer layers, which may be destroyed during the refining process.

Fat-soluble vitamins are stored in the liver, fat tissues, and muscles. Water-soluble vitamins are not stored in the body. Any excess amounts leave the body through the kidneys and urine. Therefore, they need to be consumed on a regular basis to prevent deficiency. The exception is vitamin B12, reserves of which can be stored in the liver for years.

Fat-soluble vitamins

Vitamin A: retinols and carotenoids

Vitamin A is a family of chemicals that includes retinol (derived from animal sources), and about 50 different carotenoids (pro-vitamin A, derived from plants), which are yellow or orange plant pigments found in many fruits and vegetables. The most common carotenoid is beta-carotene, which is found in abundance in carrots, green leaves, and peppers, and yellow, orange, red, and green plants. Other important carotenoids include alpha-carotene, gamma-carotene, lycopene, and cryptoxanthin. These precursors are hydrolysed and split into two molecules of vitamin A (retinol) in the cells of the intestinal wall during digestion. High-fat animal foods contain vitamin A as retinol.

By law in Britain, vitamin (as retinol or beta-carotene) is added to margarine, which is thus a major source of the vitamin for the general population.

Absorption

Vitamin A is absorbed in fat droplets or chylomicrons, from the intestinal cells where it is processed. Its absorption is increased with lecithin (an emulsifier that impacts the gut microbiota, and is found in many plant-based and animal foods, including soya and eggs).

The liver stores vitamin A in enough quantity to act as a reserve for many months. About one sixth of the carotenoids we eat are converted into retinol in the body and stored in the liver, fat tissues, lungs, testicles, bone marrow, eyes, and kidneys. Vitamin A is important for good vision, skin, reproduction, pregnancy, growth, and immunity, and it also protects against bacterial, parasitic, and viral infections. In addition, carotenoids are powerful antioxidants that help us resist cancer and heart disease.

The average adult needs about 600–700 mcg of retinol or 3300 mcg of beta-carotene per day. Vitamin A is found in many different foods, so deficiency ought to be rare in affluent societies, but during illness, and in cases of fat malabsorption, extra pro-vitamin A is needed in the diet.

Vitamin A's main functions:

- it forms part of visual pigments and helps vision, especially in dim light
- it helps the formation of tears
- it aids nuclear receptors that regulate gene expression and tissue differentiation, so it is important for cell growth, for foetal development, and for growth in children
- it is vital for hair growth
- it maintains fertility
- plant-based pro-vitamin A (carotenoid) is an antioxidant against harmful free radicals and can be used for cancer prevention and as part of a treatment protocol
- beta-carotene has an anti-tumour effect, and there may be a relationship between low dietary beta-carotene and cancer
- it helps the immune system protect us against illness and infection
- it keeps skin and mucous membranes in good health.

Deficiency

Vitamin A deficiency is a major public health problem worldwide with more than 200 million children affected due to poverty, disease, and severe shortages of fresh food. Vitamin A deficiency causes decreased immunity, and it is the commonest preventable cause of eye disease and blindness among children in developing countries.

Symptoms of vitamin A deficiency include:

- night blindness
- dry eyes
- hair loss
- skin problems—hyperkeratosis (thickening of the skin)
- poor immune function.

Taking supplements has been shown to be ineffective in the treatment of vitamin A deficiency because absorption and oxidation of carotene are limited, and significantly less retinol is absorbed than predicted.

Toxicity

Carotenoids in foods are well-absorbed, and consuming a lot of carotenoid-rich foods may tint the skin yellow. This is a completely non-toxic effect that goes away when you stop eating so much carotene.

By contrast, too much retinol can cause bone and liver damage and, in pregnancy, may harm the developing baby and cause birth defects. Signs of retinol toxicity include headache, blurred vision, vomiting, and vertigo.

More than 1500 mcg retinol per day over many years can affect your bones and can make them fracture more easily with age. This is particularly important for older women who are also susceptible to osteoporosis.

As vitamin A is stored in the liver, eating liver paté more than once per week could lead to long-term toxicity. Supplements, such as cod liver oil, are also high in retinol and should be taken with caution. Make sure your daily intake doesn't exceed 1500 mcg.

Vitamin A top ten (micrograms per 100 grams of food)

Pro-vitamin A (beta-carotene)		Retinol	
RDA = 3300 micrograms/day Toxicity level = none		RDA = 600–700 micrograms/day Acute toxicity level = acute 9000 mcg Long-term toxicity level = 1500 mcg	
	mcg/100g		mcg/100g
1. Paprika	36,250	1. Polar bear liver	900,000
2. Carrots	12,472	2. Cod liver oil	18,000
3. Sweet potato	8910	3. Lamb liver	18,100
4. Spring greens/nettle	8295	4. Beef/calf, average	15,500
5. Parsley	4040	5. Chicken/duck average	9500
6. Red pepper	3780	6. Liver paté	7300
7. Spinach	3535	7. Butter	958
8. Curly kale	3145	8. Double cream	779
9. Watercress	2520	9. Cheese	300
10. Yellow melon	1765	10. Egg	190

Source: MAFF. The Composition of Foods.

Vitamin D: ergocalciferol (D2) and cholecalciferol (D3)

At the beginning of the twentieth century, a bone disease called rickets was rife among poor children in northern industrialised countries. It was cured—and prevented—with cod liver oil, and research revealed that this effect could be reproduced by two chemicals, cholecalciferol (vitamin D3, found in animal tissues) and ergocalciferol (vitamin D2, found in plant sterols).

Vitamin D is actually a steroid hormone mainly obtained from exposure to sunlight. Bright sunshine is not necessary, and even skyshine on a cloudy day will stimulate formation of some vitamin D in the skin. A short summer holiday in the open air will increase serum levels of vitamin D two- or three-fold.

Vitamin D plays a major role in maintaining calcium blood levels and calcium uptake into cells, as well as mobilisation of calcium within cells. It also regulates cell proliferation in many body tissues, and is involved in secretion of hormones.

Many foods are now fortified with vitamin D, but sunlight is our most important source because it triggers vitamin D production in the skin. Just one hour a day of sunlight on a small patch of skin is enough, and, during the summer, the body produces and stores plenty to last the winter—unless the skin is covered by clothes or sunscreen. Around 300 cases of rickets were reported in the UK in 2014, and it is thought the reasons are excessive sunscreen use combined with children spending more time indoors than outside playing.

Vitamin D photosynthesis

Humans photosynthesise vitamin D3 in their skin by UV irradiation of 7-dehydrocholesterol, which is a precursor to cholesterol produced naturally in the liver.

The skin of animals and birds is protected from UV radiation by their fur and feathers. Instead, they produce oils and waxes that impregnate fur and feathers, making them waterproof and also producing vitamin D3 by photosynthesis. The vitamin is then ingested when they groom themselves.

When commonly eaten mushrooms, such as button mushrooms, oyster mushrooms, and shiitake mushrooms, are exposed to UV radiation, they also generate vitamin D, mainly D2, from ergosterol in the mushroom cell wall. When fresh mushrooms are deliberately exposed to midday sunlight for 15–20 minutes, they generate in excess of 10 mcg D2/100g. When fresh-harvested mushrooms are exposed to UV radiation from lamps, they can generate up to 40 mcg per 100g. Sundried mushrooms also contain an average of 16.9 mcg vitamin D2 per gram (dried weight).

Wild mushrooms, such as the funnel chanterelle, have been found to provide up to 30 mcg D2 per hundred grams, and the cep mushroom (*Boletus edulis*) was found to contain 59 mcg D2/100g.

Experiments have shown that mushrooms retain 85% of their vitamin D content after frying.

The consumption of mushrooms is growing worldwide, and since they also provide good amounts of protein, B vitamins, calcium, selenium, potassium, zinc, and copper, they are becoming important sources of nutrients. Vitamin D-enhanced mushrooms containing high concentrations of vitamin D2 are also now being produced by commercial growers. This could be an important solution for the worldwide public health concern about vitamin D deficiency.

Plants that contain sterols are also attracting interest as sources of vitamin D, and it is now known that vitamin D3 is formed in certain plants, especially the nightshade family (Solanaceae). These contain high amounts of vitamin D3—potato, tomato, and pepper plants have all been found to contain vitamin D in their leaves.

Microalgae and edible seaweed also contain a sizable amounts of vitamin D, as does lichen, which is a small unique composite organism that comes from algae or cyanobacteria living on fungi. Lichens are abundant, growing on bark, or hanging from branches, on rocks, walls, and roofs. It is estimated that there are around 20,000 species of lichen and that they are among the oldest living things on earth. Iceland moss (*Cetraria islandica*), for example, is a lichen that has been used as an important food and medicine in northern Europe.

Vitamin D is needed for the absorption and utilisation of calcium by the body, and for maintenance of normal blood calcium and phosphorus levels. It does this by enhancing the absorption of calcium from the intestine and by helping to regulate the movement of calcium between bone and blood.

Vitamin D from food or supplements is absorbed by chylomicrons in the small intestine. Secretions from the stomach, pancreas, and liver all influence absorption, as does the health of the gut wall. Therefore, problems that affect gut health and digestion, such as coeliac, Crohn's, liver disease, and pancreatitis, can all inhibit vitamin D absorption. Blood levels of vitamin D are also affected by kidney health, and people with kidney problems often suffer from vitamin D deficiency.

Deficiency

Vitamin D plays an important role in many aspects of health. In infancy and childhood, a deficiency of vitamin D causes the deformed bones characteristic of rickets. In adults, a lack of the vitamin causes osteomalacia, which is a softening of the bones.

Vitamin D deficiency also linked to:

- stunted growth
- back pain
- bone pain and deformity
- dental problems
- nerve problems

- muscle weakness
- anaemia
- anxiety and depression
- fatigue
- type 2 diabetes
- chronic inflammation
- multiple sclerosis
- heart disease
- a predisposition to respiratory infections
- and lowered immunity.

Osteoporosis is not directly caused by vitamin D deficiency, but it may be beneficial to take vitamin D as part of an osteoporosis treatment protocol.

Vitamin D deficiency is one of the most common nutritional deficiencies worldwide. Exacerbating factors include lack of exposure to sunlight.

The most common risk factors include:

- being housebound
- working overnight shifts
- being pregnant or breastfeeding
- being elderly
- following a strict religious dress code
- working as a submariner or astronaut
- living at high altitude
- having chronic kidney or liver problems
- hyperparathyroidism and parathyroid tumours
- having digestive disorders that affect absorption
- having gastric bypass surgery
- taking statins or steroids
- using sunscreen.

Toxicity

Intakes of vitamin D higher than the recommended daily amount are now thought to protect against cancer and metabolic syndrome (late-onset diabetes), but there is insufficient evidence to support this view.

An excess of vitamin D causes hypercalcaemia (high levels of calcium in the blood), and this may lead to calcium deposition in the tissues, especially the kidneys where stones can lead to renal damage and even failure. Excessive intakes of vitamin D are more dangerous for infants than for adults. Intakes of 50 micrograms per day have been associated with hypercalcaemia in children. Infants are sensitive to hypercalcaemia, and because of that, the level of fortification of baby foods is limited. The downside is that this may result in a proportion of infants being at risk of developing rickets.

Symptoms of toxicity include:

- loss of appetite
- nausea
- diarrhoea
- muscle weakness
- joint pain
- headache
- stomach ache
- cramp
- high blood pressure.

Vitamin D top ten (micrograms per 100 grams of food)

Cholecalciferol

RDA = 10 micrograms/day
Toxicity level >50 mcg/day

		mcg/100g
1.	Cod liver oil	210.0
2.	Microalgae	72.0–271.0
3.	Japanese wireweed (seaweed)	90.0
4.	Lichen	25.0
5.	Chestnut mushrooms (exposed to UV light)	31.9
6.	Herring	19.0
7.	Cod roe	17.0
8.	Salmon	16.7
9.	Trout	9.6
10.	Mackerel	8.2

Source: MAFF. The Composition of Foods.

Vitamin E: tocopherols

Vitamin E comprises eight substances called tocopherols, the most active being alpha tocopherol, which helps regulate platelet coagulation and smooth muscle formation, but they all have different biological activities and antioxidant action. Together they make up a yellow, oily liquid that is remarkably stable to heat but unstable to oxygen, alkalis, and UV light. The vitamin is found widely in foods, the richest sources being vegetable oils, nuts, whole grain, flours, and wheat germ. Meat, animal fats, fruit, and vegetables contain very little vitamin E.

Being fat-soluble, vitamin E is stored in the body and so a daily intake is not essential. This, combined with its fairly wide availability, means that deficiency is rare. There is, however, some evidence that vitamin E is essential to the normal functioning of red blood cells in both children and adults.

Vitamin E is a major antioxidant, which stabilises cell membranes and protects them against damage from free radicals and environmental toxins. It also inhibits the production of the inflammatory prostaglandins that cause many of the symptoms of autoimmune diseases such as rheumatoid arthritis. It plays a role in the synthesis of DNA, and it is thought to protect against heart disease and cancer, and it is also part of lowering blood cholesterol levels.

Deficiency

Vitamin E is found in a wide variety of foods, so deficiency is not common, but since it has important effects on immune function, there is a distinction between the amount needed to avoid dietary deficiency and the amount needed to help prevent disease. Higher intakes of up to 50 mg per day can decrease the risk of immune-related conditions and help prevent or delay the development of Parkinson's disease and other degenerative neurological disorders such as multiple sclerosis. Vitamin E is also thought to reduce the risk of cataracts, arthritis, and chronic fatigue syndrome.

Deficiency really only occurs in people with serious fat malabsorption problems, or with genetic nerve damage disorders.

Because of its role as an antioxidant and in stabilising cell membranes, vitamin E deficiency leads to cell membrane damage, which in turn causes muscle, nerve, and liver dysfunction. As tobacco smoke contains large amounts of free radicals, smokers should ensure their diet contains plenty of vitamin E, as should the elderly and people with liver disease in whom increased susceptibility to illness may be related to deficiency.

Toxicity

When obtained from food, vitamin E has no toxic effects. But taking high-dose vitamin E supplements may cause breast soreness, muscle weakness, psychological and gastrointestinal disturbance, and thyroid dysfunction.

Vitamin E top ten (milligrams per 100 grams of food)

Vitamin E—tocopherol

RDA = >4 milligrams/day
Toxicity level >540 mg/day

		mg/100g
1.	Wheat germ oil	136.7
2.	Sunflower oil	49.2
3.	Safflower oil	40.7
4.	Sunflower seeds	37.8
5.	Polyunsaturated vegetable margarine	32.6
6.	Almonds, hazelnuts	24.5
7.	Sundried tomatoes	24.0
8.	Wheat germ	22.0
9.	Corn oil	17.2
10.	Pine nuts	13.7

Source: MAFF. The Composition of Foods.

Vitamin K: phylloquinone (K1) and menaquinone (K2)

K1 is produced by plants involved in photosynthesis (those with green leaves), and K2 is produced by bacteria involved in fermentation. Intestinal bacteria also produce vitamin K, especially if we eat a high-fibre diet, but it is not known to what extent this contributes to blood levels of the vitamin, which is stored in the liver and recycled many times before being broken down and excreted.

Vitamin K plays a vital role in normal blood clotting and bone health. It may help prevent osteoporosis and protect soft tissues from abnormal calcification.

Vitamin K is widespread in plant foods, especially dark green vegetables, and also in cabbage, cauliflower, peas, and grains. It is provided in roughly equal proportions by diet and from bacterial activity in the gut.

Deficiency

Deficiency is rare, but digestive and malabsorption diseases, such as coeliac disease, pancreatitis, cystic fibrosis, and chronic liver disease, may cause deficiency since vitamin K depends on normal fat digestion for its own absorption. It can also be caused by broad-spectrum orally administered antibiotics, which destroy the normal gut flora, and anticoagulants can inhibit normal metabolism of vitamin K.

Symptoms of deficiency include:

- easy bruising and bleeding
- bone fractures.

Haemorrhagic disease of the newborn (HDN) affects a small number of babies and was shown in the 1940s to be caused by vitamin K deficiency. Newborns used to be given protective vitamin K injections, but nowadays vitamin K is given to the mother before the birth, and to the baby by mouth once it is born.

Toxicity

Natural vitamin K is non-toxic, even in large amounts. Some authorities believe that synthetic vitamin K (menadione) is less safe and better avoided.

Vitamin K top ten (micrograms per 100 grams of food)

Phylloquinone

RDA = >1 micrograms/day
Toxicity level = none

		mcg/100g
1.	Curly kale	623
2.	Parsley	548
3.	Spinach	394
4.	Watercress	315
5.	Cabbage	242
6.	Broccoli	185
7.	Brussels sprouts	153
8.	Lettuce	129
9.	Olive oil	57
10.	Asparagus	52

Source: MAFF. The Composition of Foods.

Water-soluble vitamins

The B-group vitamins

B1	–	Thiamin
B2	–	Riboflavin
B3	–	Niacin
B5	–	Pantothenate
B6	–	Pyridoxine
B7	–	Biotin
B9	–	Folate
B12	–	Cobalamin

The chemical structure of each B vitamin is different but because they have several features in common they are usually considered together as a group.

The B-vitamins are water-soluble—so don't throw away the cooking water!—and tend to be found in the same foods. They act as co-factors for enzyme systems in the body.

Intestinal bacteria synthesise considerable amounts of some B-vitamins, and in the case of folate and biotin, the gut biome may produce almost as much as we need. It has also become clear that bacterial synthesis of thiamin, riboflavin, niacin, biotin, and folate can be increased by eating fermented foods and dietary fibre.

The role of the gut biome in the synthesis and supply of these B-vitamins has largely been ignored because it was thought absorption only happens in the small intestine, whereas the biome synthesising B-vitamins occupies the large intestine. But it now turns out, and there-fore has always been the case, that specific high-affinity carrier-mediated transport systems are responsible for the absorption of the synthesised vitamins, suggesting that gut bacteria do play an important role in vitamin absorption and nutrition—another reason a healthy gut and keeping your biome happy is vital for health.

Vitamin B1: thiamin

Thiamin is a co-enzyme in metabolism and nervous system activity. We need thiamine to make use of the energy contained in carbohy-drates, fats, and alcohol, so our daily requirement is closely linked to the amount of these foods in our diet. Foods containing carbohydrate and fat usually come ready-packed with thiamine, and a diet consisting of natural, unprocessed foods normally provides all that we need. In cereals and seeds, thiamine is found in the outer grain layers and is therefore often lost during milling and refining. To remedy this loss, many processed foods are fortified with vitamin B1.

Deficiency

The more carbohydrate is consumed, the more thiamin is required. Thus if high levels of mainly refined, unfortified carbohydrates are eaten, thiamine deficiency may result. Deficiency of thiamine causes palpitations and muscular weakness, and, in severe cases, beriberi.

The three distinct symptoms of thiamin deficiency are chronic peripheral neuritis, beriberi, and Wernicke's encephalopathy (neurological symptoms caused by biochemical lesions of the central nervous system characterised by weak eye muscles, lack of coordination of muscle movement, and confusion).

Towards the end of the nineteenth century an epidemic of beriberi spread through Japan, China, and Southeast Asia, causing serious problems for the colonial powers with their insatiable need for cheap labour. Mortality rates exceeded 50% and, although it was noticed that the disease could be cured by supplementing the staple diet of rice with fish, vegetables, meat, and grains, poverty ensured that the epidemic continued. The cause of the beriberi only emerged when an "anti-beriberi-factor" (thiamin) was discovered in rice polishings—the parts of the rice grain removed during dehulling to produce polished white rice. The introduction of steam-powered mills and the production of polished rice on an industrial scale had robbed the rice grain of its nutrients, and the labourers who produced it of their health.

Nowadays, vitamin B1 deficiency is often associated with alcoholism, malnutrition, and chronic disease. It is a significant underdiagnosed problem among alcoholics, drug users, and HIV AIDS sufferers. When deficiency becomes severe, beriberi develops, causing muscle weakness, nerve problems, and eventually heart failure. Wernicke's encephalopathy with Korsakoff's psychosis is especially linked to alcoholism, drug problems, and HIV AIDS; symptoms include confusion, loss of memory and balance, loss of muscle coordination, and visual problems such as rapid eye movement and double vision. Korsakoff's syndrome is the result of permanent brain damage.

There are two types of beriberi: wet and dry. Wet beriberi damages heart and circulation and may end in heart failure. Dry beriberi causes nerve damage and can lead to weakened muscles and, if untreated, muscle paralysis.

Toxicity

Very high doses of thiamine (>3g/day), and more moderate doses (>50 mg/day) taken over long periods, can cause toxicity symptoms such as headaches, irritability, itching, eczema, fast pulse, sleeplessness, and weakness.

Vitamin B1 —thiamin

RDA = 0.8–1 milligrams/day • Toxicity level > 3g/day

		mg/100g
1.	Quorn	36.6
2.	Yeast extract (marmite)	4.1
3.	Wheat germ	2.0
4.	Sunflower seeds	1.6
5.	Breakfast cereals	1.2
6.	Peanuts	1.1
7.	Brazil nuts	1.0
8.	Wheat bran, sesame, poppy seeds	0.9
9.	Peas	0.7
10.	Brown rice	0.6

Vitamin B2: riboflavin

Like thiamine, riboflavin has a central role as a co-enzyme used by the body for the utilisation of energy from food. In the body, riboflavin is central to all metabolic processes, including oxidation of fatty acids, and riboflavin metabolism is a main source of oxygen radicals in the body.

Cooking can destroy 30–40% of the riboflavin in vegetables, but this loss is mitigated by the riboflavin synthesised by the gut biome. There is also a very efficient conservation and recycling of riboflavin by body tissues in times of deficiency.

Most of the riboflavin in foods occurs as flavin co-enzymes bound to enzymes. Riboflavin is not well stored by the body, so the amount we need each day is related to how much food we eat, and how many calories we spend. However much riboflavin we consume, the body only uses as much as it needs, excreting the rest in the urine. It has an intense yellow colour, which is also used as a food colour, E-101, and it colours urine bright yellow when riboflavin is taken as a food supplement.

Deficiency

Mild riboflavin deficiency is relatively common, but there is no clear deficiency disease, and it is masked by the body recycling most of the riboflavin used as a co-enzyme.

People suffering from thyroid problems, diabetes, anorexia nervosa, severe malnutrition, and malabsorption syndromes may become deficient. Alcohol and some drugs, including phenothiazines (anti-psychotic medication), tricyclic antidepressants, antimalarials, and doxorubicin (a chemotherapy drug), can also reduce vitamin B2 levels in the body.

Clinically, the symptoms of deficiency include cracks at the corners of the mouth (angular stomatitis), a sore tongue that becomes red and dry ('magenta tongue'), a rash around the nose, and sometimes also a gritty feeling in the eyes (conjunctivitis) and photophobia.

B2 deficiency is also associated with hypochromic anaemia (where the red blood cells are paler than normal) as a result of iron deficiency caused by impaired iron absorption and increased loss from the gut due to lack of B2.

B3 and B6 deficiency can also be related to lack of B2.

Riboflavin deficiency in infancy and childhood (ariboflavinosis) leads to retarded growth.

Toxicity

No toxic level of riboflavin has been observed from food sources or supplements because it is only absorbed in limited amounts at any one time. Any excess is quickly excreted in the urine.

Vitamin B2—riboflavin

RDA = 1.3 mg/day for men, 1.1 mg/day for women
Toxicity level = none known

		mg/100g
1.	Yeast extract	11.90
2.	Liver, heart, kidney (average)	2.50
3.	Seaweed, nori	1.34
4.	Fortified cereals	1.20
5.	Cod roe	1.00
6.	Almonds	0.92
7.	Wheat germ	0.72
8.	Venison, duck, goose	0.60
9.	Tempeh	0.48
10.	Mushrooms	0.40

Vitamin B3: niacin

Nicotine, nicotinic acid and nicotinamide are known collectively as niacin. The niacin compounds form parts of co-enzymes involved in the release of energy. Requirements are therefore related to energy needs.

In addition to the preformed vitamin occurring in foods, one of the essential amino acids, tryptophan, may be converted in the body to niacin: 1 mg of niacin is equal to 60 mg of tryptophan. Pregnant women convert tryptophan to niacin about twice as efficiently as other people.

Apart from helping to maintain energy levels, vitamin B3 is also involved in keeping skin and mucous membranes in good condition.

Deficiency

Deficiency is rare and is usually only seen in cases of severe malnourishment or in people subsisting on foods low in niacin and tryptophan, such as maize or millet. It also affects alcoholics and cancer sufferers, and can be caused by a genetic defect.

Symptoms of niacin deficiency—also known as pellagra—include a red skin rash, sore tongue, constipation or diarrhoea, weakness, insomnia, dementia, and mental disturbance.

While pellagra responds rapidly to treatment with niacin, there is no evidence that increased intake of the vitamin is of any benefit to people without the disease.

Toxicity

There is no evidence that very large amounts of niacin produce any additional benefit for healthy people.

High doses can cause low blood pressure, flushing, and excess stomach acid. Very high doses may also cause liver damage.

Pharmacological doses of nicotinic acid (but not nicotinamide) can cause burning sensations in the face and hands. Doses in excess of 20 mg per day may cause dilation of blood vessels in the skin, but this effect wears off after a few days. Very high doses—3–6 grams per day—of nicotinic acid may cause liver damage.

Vitamin B3—Niacin

RDA = 16.5 mg/day for men, 13.2 mg/day for women
Toxicity level >3g/day

		mg/100g
1.	Yeast extract	71.0
2.	Wheat bran	32.6
3.	Peanuts	21.3
4.	Liver	19.4
5.	Paprika	18.4
6.	Breakfast cereals	15.0
7.	Game	12.0
8.	Mackerel and chicken	11.6
9.	Sesame and fennel seeds	10.4
10.	Wheat germ	9.8

Vitamin B5: pantothenate

Pantothenic means "that which is everywhere", and pantothenate, or pantothenic acid, is indeed present in almost all living tissues. It is found in most natural foods, and it is produced by bacteria in the intestine. This vitamin enables the body to utilise the energy contained in fats, carbohydrates, protein, and alcohol.

Vitamin B5 aids antibody production, protects against allergy and hypertension, and maintains nervous system health. It is also a constituent of the co-enzyme needed to convert cholesterol into steroid hormones, and in the detoxification of drugs.

It is closely associated with the adrenal glands and with our ability to respond to stress, so it is also called "the stress vitamin". An increased intake is needed in high-stress situations, after antibiotic therapy, and in allergic states.

B5 has been used in the management of rheumatoid arthritis with variable success, and as there are many reasons why rheumatoid arthritis affects people, it is good to rule out B5 deficiency as a possible cause of symptoms.

Interestingly, research has shown that the ageing process may be linked to the stress response, and that older people have lower blood levels of pantothenate than younger people.

Deficiency

Deficiency is rare because pantothenic acid is widespread in common foods and substantial amounts are produced by intestinal bacteria. It is destroyed by dry-processing of food and during roasting of meat.

Deficiency is unlikely in people who eat a diet consisting mainly of fresh foods, but in affluent societies—where many people exist on refined, canned or frozen foods, white bread, and ready-made processed meals—sub-clinical pantothenate deficiency is becoming more common.

Symptoms include weakness, insomnia, cramps, and an increased tendency to allergy. Severe deficiency is very rare and causes pins and needles, a sensation of burning in the feet, low blood pressure, and inability of the adrenal glands to respond to stress.

Toxicity

High intakes of pantothenic acid are not dangerous.

Vitamin B5—pantothenate

There is no RDA for B5 in the UK. Current intakes are 3–7 mg per day.
The WHO RDA = 5 mg/day
Toxicity level = none

		mg/100g
1.	Liver, average	6.98
2.	Broad beans	4.94
3.	Breakfast cereals, average	3.80
4.	Peanuts	2.70
5.	Cod roe	2.60
6.	Wheat germ, wheat bran	2.20
7.	Sesame seeds	2.10
8.	Mushrooms	2.00
9.	Mung beans	1.91
10.	Eggs	1.80

Vitamin B6: pyridoxine

Vitamin B6 is a mixture of six compounds that are interconvertible. Plants synthesise pyridoxine to protect themselves from ultraviolet radiation from the sun, and as part of chlorophyll synthesis. Although vitamin B6 is synthesised by bacteria in the large intestine, the amount absorbed is not sufficient to meet the needs of the host, partly because the vitamin is used by other gut bacteria. Animals must therefore obtain it from their diet, either directly from plants or other animals.

The vitamin B6 in plants is more stable than the forms found in animal-based foods, so less is lost during processing.

The more protein we eat, the more vitamin B6 we need because it is involved in protein metabolism and is necessary for the metabolism of amino acids, including conversion of tryptophan into niacin. Vitamin B6 also facilitates haemoglobin production and protects against high blood pressure and allergy. It supports the nervous system and the immune system and is used to treat nausea in early pregnancy and during radiotherapy treatment. It is also used to treat ginkgo seed poisoning, the symptoms of which include vomiting and convulsions.

Deficiency

Vitamin B6 deficiency is not common but the likelihood increases with age. It is associated with alcoholism, chronic liver and kidney disease, intestinal malabsorption disorders, and certain genetic disorders. It may also be linked to epilepsy, anaemia, and carpal tunnel syndrome, and it can also be caused by the drugs used in the treatment of tuberculosis, rheumatoid arthritis, and Parkinson's disease.

Mild deficiency in otherwise healthy people may diminish the immune response and increase the risk of atherosclerosis and hormone-dependent cancers. Deficiency may also be related to asthma, and kidney stones.

Vitamin B6 is closely involved in hormone metabolism and the menstrual cycle. Sub-clinical deficiency is relatively common in women during childbearing years, especially those who have had several pregnancies or who use oral contraceptives or HRT. Premenstrual mood swings, acne, and morning sickness—even pre-eclmapsia and post-natal depression—may be related to vitamin B6 deficiency.

Other symptoms include a skin rash around the eyes, nose and mouth cracks in the corners of the mouth and the lips, a sore tongue, migraine, depression, irritability, tiredness, and disturbed sensation in hands and feet.

Toxicity

Higher than normal intakes may help counter some of the undesirable effects of the contraceptive pill in some women, but oral contraceptives do not increase requirements for the vitamin per se.

Taking regular high doses (>50 mg/day) of vitamin B6 over a long period of time can cause toxicity. High intakes can be dangerous because this can cause loss of sensation in hands and feet, which returns once the intake is reduced. Interestingly, vitamin B6 is used to treat the common side effect of antibiotics taken for tuberculosis, which cause numbness in hands and feet.

Vitamin B6—pyridoxine

RDA in the UK = 1.4 mg/day for men, 1.2 mg/day for women
Toxicity level >200 mg/day

		mg/100g
1.	Brewer's yeast	4.2
2.	Wheat germ	3.3
3.	Tempeh	1.9
4.	Wheat bran	1.4
5.	Yeast extract	1.3
6.	Lentils	0.9
7.	Sesame seeds	0.8
8.	Oat flakes and salmon	0.7
9.	Walnuts, venison and turkey	0.6
10.	Chickpeas	0.5

Vitamin B7: biotin

Also known as Vitamin H, biotin is widely available in many foods, especially yeast. Plants synthesise biotin, and it is also synthesised by bacteria in the intestinal flora and absorbed in the colon.

Biotin functions as a co-enzyme required for the normal metabolism of fat and for a wide variety of metabolic reactions. Like the other B-group vitamins, it is needed to produce energy from carbohydrates, fats, and proteins. It is essential for healthy skin, hair, sweat glands, nerves, bone marrow, and sex glands. It also encourages appetite and aids fat metabolism.

Only very small amounts of vitamin B7 are necessary, but increased intakes may be beneficial during antibiotic therapy and during periods of stress. Biotin is also used therapeutically in the treatment of skin complaints, seborrheic dermatitis, dandruff, hair loss, and brittle nails. High-dose biotin (300 mg/day) may help promote remyelination of nerve cells to slow or reverse the neurodegeneration in multiple sclerosis.

Deficiency

Biotin deficiency is rare but can be caused by poor nutrition, and by eating large amounts of raw eggs, since raw egg white contains avidin, which combines with biotin and makes it unavailable to the body. It is also worth noting that large amounts of biotin are lost during drying of milk for formula baby foods, and cradle cap can be treated with biotin.

Symptoms of deficiency include dry skin, hair loss, fatigue, nausea, and lack of appetite.

Severe deficiency causes muscle pains, pins and needles, anaemia, and raised blood cholesterol.

Toxicity

No cases of toxicity have been reported even with very high intakes from supplements (<300 mg/day). However, high intakes of biotin, from supplements, can create false lab test results, such as false positives in lab tests for thyroid problems.

Vitamin B7 — biotin

RDA in the UK = 30 mcg/day
Toxicity level = none

		mcg/100g
1.	Chicken liver	216
2.	Dried yeast	200
3.	Peanuts	100
4.	Hazelnuts, almonds, soya beans	65
5.	Tempeh	53
6.	Plaice	47
7.	Wheat bran and wheat germ	35
8.	Eggs	25
9.	Oatmeal and oatcakes	20
10.	Mushrooms	15

Vitamin B9: folate and folic acid

As the name suggests, folate comes mainly from foliage, as it was first extracted from spinach leaves. It is found in small amounts in many leafy greens and yeasts, and most people can get enough folate from their diet. It is not stored in the body, so it needs to be a regular part of the diet.

Folate, also called folic acid, is used by the body to produce red blood cells, amino acids, and DNA. Together with vitamin B12, it supports rapidly dividing cells and is vitally important during pregnancy for the development of the baby's nervous system.

Low folate in the diet has been linked to heart disease and birth defects called neural tube defects, such as spina bifida, in unborn babies.

If you are pregnant or could get pregnant, it is recommended to take 400 mcg folic acid daily until you are 12 weeks pregnant. Folic acid levels need to be adequate before you get pregnant to help prevent neural tube defects in your baby.

Deficiency

Folate deficiency has three main causes: malnourishment, particularly among the elderly, the poor, and alcoholics, but also increasingly in people whose diet consists mainly of fast foods; malabsorption caused by gastrointestinal disease and some drugs (particularly anti-epileptic medication); and increased need, owing to pregnancy, blood disorders, blood loss, cancer, AIDS, and serious infection.

The symptoms of deficiency include weakness, depression, and macrocytic anaemia. In fact, in the 1920s, scientists thought that folate deficiency and anaemia were the same condition.

Toxicity

Very high intakes of vitamin B9, usually from supplements, are not toxic but can lead to reduced zinc absorption. Taking more than 1 mg per day can mask symptoms of vitamin B12 deficiency. This is particularly a problem for older people because it becomes more difficult to absorb vitamin B12 with age.

Vitamin B9—folic acid and folate

RDA in the UK = 200 mcg/day
Toxicity level = 1 mg/day

		mcg/100g
1.	Brewer's yeast and yeast extract	2620
2.	Black-eye and pinto beans	630
3.	Chicken and calf liver	590
4.	Soya beans	370
5.	Wheat bran	260
6.	Purple sprouting broccoli	195
7.	Chickpeas	180
8.	Asparagus	175
9.	Spinach, parsley, Swiss chard	165
10.	Beetroot, savoy cabbage, sweetcorn	150

Vitamin B12: cobalamin

Vitamin B12 is the most complex of all vitamins. It is, in fact, a mixture of related compounds, all containing cobalt—hence the name "cobalamin". It is produced entirely by microorganisms, not by plants, nor by animals directly, but by their gut biome. It can be found in soil, manure, and unsanitised water, and also in yeast extract, nori seaweed, and shiitake mushrooms. Many plant-based foods are fortified with vitamin B12.

Microorganisms in the gut biome of humans and other animals make vitamin B12. There is also evidence that the microflora in the small intestine synthesise significant amounts of cobalamin. The absorption of B12 in the small intestine requires intrinsic factor produced by the stomach. The absorption is aided by calcium. What isn't absorbed is excreted in the faeces, and human and animal faeces contain vitamin B12 produced by bacteria in the colon. Some animals eat their faeces as a B12 supplement, and trials with giving humans extracts of their own faeces as supplements have been successful in correcting deficiency.

It is worth noting that farm animals are also routinely fed vitamin B12 supplements in their diet, sometimes in the form of dried excrement.

Vitamin B12 is used in DNA synthesis and is essential for all body cells, particularly blood and nerve cells. Rapidly dividing cells in the bone marrow need vitamin B12 and folic acid to produce red and white blood cells. It is also used to release energy from the food we eat, and to help the body use folate.

Only tiny amounts are needed, and it is stored in the liver, which normally contains enough to sustain the body for 3–6 years. It is excreted in the bile and then reabsorbed. At low dietary levels, there is a high absorption rate from the small intestine.

Deficiency

Malabsorption syndromes, intestinal parasites, gastrointestinal ulcers, alcoholism, and cancer are the most likely causes of deficiency. Smoking and taking antibiotics also increase need. Vegans should include non-animal B12 sources or supplements in their diet.

Symptoms of deficiency include a sore tongue, diarrhoea, and general weakness, progressing to numbness and tingling in fingers and toes, loss of balance, nerve pains, and weakness in arms and legs caused by damage to the spinal cord and brain.

Pernicious anaemia is a rare form of vitamin B12 deficiency caused by a lack of "intrinsic factor", which is a protein secretion in the stomach. Without intrinsic factor, B12 cannot be absorbed.

Vitamin B12 deficiency is also associated with dementia, but there is no evidence that taking supplements can help prevent or treat dementia.

People suffering from malabsorption syndromes, including pernicious anaemia, usually need vitamin B12 injections.

Some drugs, including amino-salicylic acid, colchicine, metformin, proton pump inhibitors, and vitamin C supplements, may inhibit B12 absorption.

Toxicity

Vitamin B12 is non-toxic, even in large doses, but taking high doses can cause headache, nausea and vomiting, diarrhoea, fatigue or weakness, and tingling sensations in hands and feet.

Vitamin B12—cobalamin

RDA in the UK = 1.5 mcg/day
Toxicity level = 2 mg

		mcg/100g
1.	Liver	58
2.	Tartex (fortified bean paste)	50
3.	Cockles, mussels	35
4.	Nori seaweed	28
5.	Sardines	25
6.	Yeast extract	13
7.	Mackerel	10
8.	Prawns, herring, salmon, trout	6
9.	Vegetable margarine (fortified)	5
10.	Meat and eggs, average	3

Vitamin C: ascorbic acid

Vitamin C is important for human health, being needed for many physiological functions in the body, particularly for maintaining healthy connective tissue, skin, blood vessels, bones, and cartilage. It is essential for collagen, carnitine, and neurotransmitter synthesis.

As it is a water-soluble vitamin, vitamin C is easily absorbed but not stored in the body. The average adult has a body pool of 1.2–2 grams of ascorbic acid, which may be maintained with 40 mg of the vitamin from food per day. The pool is usually depleted in 4–12 weeks if no vitamin C is eaten in the diet or taken as a supplement.

In nature, vitamin C is found in association with vitamin P (bioflavonoids and rutin). The best sources of vitamin C are fresh fruit and vegetables, including potatoes. It is damaged by cooking and food processing, and is lost in cooking water. Freeze drying preserves ascorbic acid.

Vitamin C is an important antioxidant and plays a vital role in wound healing and iron absorption. It stimulates immune system cells to fight infections and helps lower blood cholesterol. It also reduces the toxic effects of radiation and protects against serious diseases such as cancer and heart disease.

As an antioxidant, it helps avoid oxidative damage, which is implicated in chronic disease such as cardiovascular disease, stroke, cancer, neurodegenerative disorders, and cataract. There is compelling evidence that ascorbic acid inhibits LDL oxidation and therefore also the formation of atherosclerosis.

Vitamin C promotes iron absorption and storage in bone marrow, spleen, and liver. It is involved in the production of collagen, in the immune response, in the control of blood cholesterol levels, in the production of anti-stress hormones, in normal brain function, in tooth and bone formation, in keeping blood vessels and sex organs healthy, and in the actions of folic acid and vitamin E. It also has some antihistamine properties.

Unlike most animals, humans and apes are unable to synthesise vitamin C from glucose, so we have to include it in our diet. Current recommended daily amounts are based on the amount necessary to protect against scurvy and promote wound healing, but many people could benefit from eating more. Animals that synthesise their own have much higher body levels of vitamin C than most humans, so it has been suggested that our vitamin C intake should be increased to produce similar levels. Cancer and rheumatoid arthritis sufferers have decreased amounts of vitamin C in their blood, as do smokers. Stress, infection, and burns also deplete vitamin C reserves in the body, which demands higher doses of the vitamin in the diet or as a supplement.

Deficiency

Deficiency results in bleeding, especially from small blood vessels, such as gums. It also causes slow wound healing. Mild deficiency may occur in infants who are given unsupplemented cow's milk, in people eating poor diets, as for example the elderly, and in people eating insufficient fresh fruit and vegetables.

Severe deficiency produces scurvy.

In the eighteenth century, scurvy was much feared by seafarers. The first signs were bleeding gums, leg pains, slow-healing wounds, and general weakness, followed by haemorrhages under the skin, swellings, ulcers, and death. In 1772, James Lind (a Scottish physician) found that including citrus fruit in seamen's diets would cure scurvy in a week. Subsequent research showed that ascorbic acid, now known as vitamin C, was the key, and it is now known that 10 mg ascorbic acid per day is sufficient to prevent and cure all signs of scurvy.

Toxicity

Today, scurvy appears only in cases of famine, severe malnutrition, malabsorption, and chronic alcoholism. However, people who take more than one gram of vitamin C supplements per day can develop signs of scurvy if they suddenly reduce their intake—even though their diet provides the recommended daily amount. Very high intakes of vitamin C can cause diarrhoea and increase the risk of kidney stones.

Intakes of twenty times the RDA or more have been associated with diarrhoea and an increased risk of developing oxalate kidney stones. Supplementation with ascorbic acid should thus be avoided in cases of urinary tract stones and if urate levels are high, such as in gout. Precipitation of urate and cystine stones is more likely in the presence of high levels of vitamin C.

Taking more than 1 gram per day can cause stomach pain, diarrhoea, and wind.

Vitamin C—ascorbic acid

RDA = 40 milligrams/day
Toxicity level >1000 mg/day

		mg/100g
1.	Guava	230
2.	Chilli peppers	225
3.	Blackcurrants	200
4.	Parsley	190
5.	Spring greens	180
6.	Redcurrants	140
7.	Red and green peppers	130
8.	Horseradish	120
9.	Brussels sprouts	115
10.	Curly kale/purple sprouting broccoli	110

In comparison, oranges and lemon only contain 50 mg vitamin C per 100g.

Source: MAFF. The Composition of Foods.

CHAPTER 11

All about major minerals and trace elements

Minerals are naturally occurring substances with distinctive chemical and physical properties, compositions, and structures. They are solid chemical compounds with a special natural crystal structure. They form part of the earth and of the human body, where they are necessary for building strong bones and teeth, controlling the movement of fluids in and out of cells, and for turning food into energy. In fact, minerals play essential roles in many different body functions, and getting too much or too little can upset delicate body balances.

Key minerals for human health are classified into major minerals and trace elements, and there are 16 in all. Major minerals are used and stored in large quantities in the body. Trace elements are just as important for health at the major minerals, but they are only needed in minute amounts.

All the essential minerals come from rocks, soil, and water; we can't make them ourselves. They are absorbed by plants and passed on to people and animals as they eat the plants.

If your diet is rich in unprocessed plant foods, it is hard to avoid getting enough minerals. Calcium is an example of a mineral people are concerned about getting enough of, and so are iron, magnesium, and potassium; but as you will see from the following tables, plants provide enough of them to cover your need—if you eat enough plants! Imbalances accompanied by a need for supplementation only arise when your diet is based more on manmade foods.

There are seven major minerals:

Calcium (Ca)
Chloride (Cl)
Magnesium (Mg)
Phosphorus (P)
Potassium (K)
Sodium (Na)
Sulphur (S)

There are nine trace elements:

Chromium (Cr)
Copper (Cu)
Fluoride (F)
Iodine (I)
Iron (Fe)
Manganese (Mn)
Molybdenum (Mo)
Selenium (Se)
Zinc (Zn)

As the amount of each mineral you need at any given point can be quite precise, they are most efficient when they come from food, and it is very difficult to overdose on minerals from foods because the body only absorbs what it needs at the time. Iron supplements, for example, can make you constipated, and can also upset your body's natural ability to regulate iron, which in turn creates too many free radicals that may contribute to heart problems and liver disease. Another example is taking too many calcium supplements, which can be linked to kidney stones and cardiovascular problems.

Absorption of minerals

The body finds absorption of dietary minerals relatively difficult. Under normal circumstances, fats, carbohydrates, proteins, and vitamins are assumed to be absorbed 100%, but most minerals average only 10–15% absorption. Exceptions are the simple mineral ions like Na+ (sodium), K+ (potassium), and Cl- (chloride), which are completely absorbed.

The intestinal tract exerts some control over the amount of minerals absorbed, and this in turn depends on body status of each mineral.

Minerals cannot be destroyed (unlike vitamins), but they can be removed by the processing and refining of foods. They can also be rendered insoluble and unavailable for absorption by other constituents of the diet.

All minerals are obtained from the soil in which the plants grow. Thus, any deficiency in the soil will be reflected in the mineral content of the plants. In fact, herbalists used to potentise yellow dock root (*Rumex crispus*) with iron by burying iron nails next to it. Yellow dock has an affinity for absorbing iron, and it is an excellent gentle laxative, which counters the constipating effect of the iron content.

Over the past decades we have seen a growth in the use of vitamins taken in high dosages for their therapeutic effect. This approach is largely ineffective with minerals. If large amounts are taken, the body simply rejects the excess. Unabsorbed minerals may cause problems in the gastrointestinal tract—as mentioned, excess iron causes stomach pain, colic, and constipation.

It is interesting to note that the mineral elements, as well as the vitamins, are found in greatest abundance in the dark layers and covering of cereals and rice, and in the rinds of fruit and vegetables.

Functions of minerals

1. Constituents of bones and teeth (calcium, phosphorus, and magnesium).
2. Soluble salts helping to regulate the electrical and osmotic composition of body fluids and cells (sodium and chloride in the extracellular fluid surrounding body cells, and potassium, magnesium, and phosphorus in the intracellular fluid inside body cells).
3. Essential adjuncts to many enzymes and other proteins that are necessary for the release and utilisation of energy. Most minerals act in this way. They are also involved in the normal functioning of many vitamins.

Major minerals

Calcium

Calcium is the most abundant mineral in the body. In association with silicon, phosphorus, and magnesium, it comprises over 50% of the bony structure of the body and gives tensile strength to body tissues.

All but 1% of calcium in the body is bound in bones and teeth. The remaining 1% is used in muscle contraction—including the heart—in nerve conduction, and in various other enzyme systems and blood clotting. Apart from giving strength to bones, calcium is constantly withdrawn into and replaced from the blood at carefully controlled rates according to need.

The skeleton acts like a calcium bank, ensuring that there is always enough calcium available in the bloodstream to support vital functions. Deposits and withdrawals are controlled by hormones, including parathyroid and thyroid hormones, calcitonin, growth hormone, sex hormones, stress hormones, and insulin. If dietary calcium is lacking, or there is a problem with absorption, the calcium bank account may become overdrawn, causing problems such as tooth decay, osteoporosis, osteomalacia, and rickets.

It is thought-provoking to reflect over whether older people break their hip because they fall, of whether they fall because their hip becomes so decalcified that it can no longer carry their weight. I once saw an old man suddenly fall in a corridor because his hip gave way. It was clear that the fall was caused by the head of femur breaking, not the other way around.

Absorption and excretion

Calcium absorption from food depends on the presence of vitamin D, and it is influenced by lifestyle choices including diet, alcohol intake, smoking, and exercise.

The amount absorbed depends on availability and how much is circulating in the blood. The normal absorption rate from a healthy diet is between 20 and 35%. Without adequate amounts of vitamin D, little or no calcium is absorbed. Oxalate and phytate from some plant foods may inhibit calcium absorption.

Plant foods such as leafy greens contain less calcium than dairy products but they have a higher bioavailability than dairy. Tofu has the same bioavailability as milk, while the biovavailability of calcium from almonds is only around 20%.

Although spinach is very high in calcium, as are all greens, the oxalate content of spinach lowers its bioavailability to only 5%. That doesn't mean you should stop eating spinach but only that you can't rely on spinach as a calcium supplement despite its very high calcium content, and it is worth remembering that the oxalate in spinach does not inhibit calcium absorption from other foods.

High calcium intakes are sometimes recommended for osteoporosis, but there is no firm evidence that this is effective without also correcting other health issues and imbalances such as getting enough exercise, vitamin D, keeping your caffeine intake down, limiting salt intake and increasing your potassium and phosphorus intake, genetic factors. There is evidence that changing your protein intake from animal-based to plant-based protein decreased calcium loss in the urine.

Calcium is excreted via the kidneys in the urine and via the skin as sweat.

Calcium deficiency

Deficiency in young children leads to rickets, which is softening of the bones caused by impaired bone metabolism or by resabsorption of calcium. If it happens in adults, it is called osteomalacia.

Old people, especially women, often suffer from osteoporosis, which is loss of bone mass and deterioration of bone tissue. It has become endemic in the UK and the US, and some authorities link osteoporosis with long-standing nutritional calcium deficiency.

However, actual deficiency of calcium in the diet is uncommon because the body will adapt to low intakes by increasing absorption. Among the Bantu peoples in Africa, whose diet is low in dairy and animal protein and high in phytate, very few eat as much as 500 mg calcium per day, and the women have an average of six children that they breastfeed. The typical Bantu diet consists of mainly of maize, beans, sorghum, vegetables, and fruits, with very little dairy and animal protein. Yet osteoporosis is rare—only 1 in 200 suffer from the disease.

In Scandinavia, where people consume plenty of dairy products and animal protein, one in two women and one in four men suffer a fracture due to osteoporosis at some point in their lives. Comparing bone mineral masses in elderly Caucasian women show that vegetarians have significantly higher bone mass than omnivores.

Osteoporosis in menopausal women is often treated with oestrogen supplementation to help preserve calcium balance but a high supplemented intake of calcium as a treatment for osteoporosis seems more or less ineffective.

Toxicity

Increased intakes of calcium lead to reduced absorption, but accumulation of calcium may be caused by failure in the body's control mechanism, rather than by high intake.

Too much calcium in the bloodstream—usually the result of excessive calcium supplements or indigestion remedies—causes nausea, depression, and even kidney stones and kidney damage.

High intakes of calcium may also reduce the absorption of other minerals and trace elements, especially iron, but there is no clear evidence that this is the case.

Hypercalcemia is a condition where blood calcium levels are above normal. This can weaken bones, create kidney stones and interfere with the function of the heart and brain. It is usually caused by overactive parathyroid glands, or by kidney failure, adrenal insufficiency, cancer, tuberculosis, sarcoidosis, Paget's disease, or some medications (such as antacids), or by taking too many calcium or vitamin A or D supplements.

Calcium (Ca)

RDA in the UK = 700 mg/day
Toxicity level = not defined
The average Brit gets 75 mg calcium/day in "hard water"

		mg/100g
1.	Baking powder	11,300
2.	Parmesan cheese	1025
3.	Seaweed (wakame, kombu, nori)	430–900
4.	Spinach	588
5.	Tofu	510
6.	Cheese (on average)	450
7.	Anchovies and sardines	420
8.	Parsley	333
9.	Figs, almonds, watercress	250
10.	Spring greens, broccoli, curly kale	200

Magnesium

Magnesium is found in most foods and, after calcium, is the second most abundant mineral in the body. It is present in bone and teeth, and is an essential constituent of all cells. It is necessary for the proper functioning of enzyme systems involved in energy utilisation, and it is also essential for efficient utilisation of vitamin B1 in releasing energy from alcohol and fats, and vitamin B6 in the metabolism of protein.

It also enhances calcium absorption and retention in the body, but excess calcium suppresses magnesium absorption. Magnesium promotes the deposition of calcium in bone and its removal from soft tissues. It is an essential constituent of chlorophyll and is thus abundant in vegetables. Less than half of dietary magnesium is normally absorbed and, unlike calcium, the process is not affected by vitamin D.

Magnesium helps to maintain healthy bones and teeth, and it protects against epilepsy, hypertension, heart disease, osteoporosis, premenstrual tension, and mental disturbance. It is used in the treatment of high blood pressure during pregnancy and as an anticonvulsant, and to calm palpitations.

Magnesium is important for the parathyroid glands to work normally, and it is also the main ingredient in many antacids and laxatives. It is difficult to say how much dietary magnesium is necessary because the body only absorbs what it needs at any given time, regardless of availability. If dietary magnesium is low, absorption becomes more efficient, and less is excreted by the kidneys, in order to maintain the right magnesium levels in the blood.

Deficiency

Deficiency is rare because magnesium is abundant in food. But it sometimes occurs as a result of excess loss in severe diarrhoea. A diet high in processed and refined foods may be deficient in magnesium, and deficiency is also associated with kidney disease, Crohn's disease and other malabsorption syndromes, parathyroid problems, diabetes, alcoholism, and old age.

Medications can also deplete magnesium levels:

- Proton pump inhibitors (PPIs—including lansoprazole and omeprazole) used to treat acid reflux can also cause magnesium deficiency
- Diuretics (loop diuretic including furosemide, bumetanide, torsemide, ethacrynic acid, and thiazide diuretics including metolazone)
- Insulin and insulin mimetic drugs
- Antibiotics
- Antiviral medication
- Antifungals
- Beta adrenergic agonists (such as theophylline)
- Bisphosphonates
- Cardiac glycosides (Digoxin)
- Chemotherapy (amsacrine, cisplatin)
- Immunosuppressants.

Toxicity

Excess dietary magnesium may cause diarrhoea, but magnesium toxicity is rare and usually only occurs in cases of kidney failure. The first signs of toxicity are thirst and flushing, followed by falling blood pressure.

Magnesium (Mg)

RDA in the UK = 300 mg/day for men
270 mg/day for women
Toxicity level = not defined but more than 400 mg can cause diarrhoea

		mg/100g
1.	Seaweed (average)	550
2.	Wheat bran	520
3.	Culinary herbs and seeds (average)	410
4.	Brazil nuts	400
5.	Sesame and sunflower seeds	380
6.	Almonds, cashews, pine nuts	270
7.	Wholemeal bread	230
8.	Beans and chickpeas	170
9.	Walnuts, amaranth leaves	130
10.	Swiss chard, spinach, okra, kale	75

Phosphorus

Phosphorus is the third most abundant mineral in the body. Calcium-phosphates are found in bones and teeth. Inorganic phosphorus is found in body cells. Phosphorus plays an essential role in the liberation and utilisation of energy from food.

All living beings use ATP as an energy source and for cell communication and DNA synthesis. So, phosphorus is an essential mineral and energy facilitator. Phosphorus is a constituent of nucleic acids and some fats, proteins, and carbohydrates, and it is therefore present in all foods.

A proper balance between phosphorus and calcium in the body is necessary for health. The kidneys, bones, and intestines regulate blood phosphorus levels very closely by blocking absorption or increasing excretion. The kidneys play a central role in maintaining this balance by controlling the amount of phosphorus lost in the urine. However, it is also important to balance phosphorus and calcium in the diet, particularly for children and infants who have smaller and more sensitive bodies than adults—too much phosphorus in a baby's diet (for example from unprocessed cow's milk) can cause muscle spasms. Excess phosphorus inhibits absorption of calcium and magnesium. Many soft drinks, processed foods, and some food additives contain inorganic phosphorus to preserve colour, moisture, and texture. Inorganic phosphorus is very easily absorbed and provides up to 30% of phosphorus intake in the normal Western diet.

Deficiency

Phosphorus deficiency is called hypophosphatemia and is very rare because phosphorus is present in nearly all foods, but pregnancy, vitamin D deficiency, serious injury, chronic gastrointestinal malabsorption syndromes, cancer, liver disease, anorexia, uncontrolled diabetes, some drugs, and alcoholism can all cause phosphorus levels to fall. This can cause demineralisation of bones, lower immunity, and may lead to muscle weakness and softening of the bones (osteomalacia).

Symptoms of phosphorus deficiency include poor appetite, bone pain, confusion, muscle weakness, increased susceptibility to infection, and anaemia. In children, deficiency may cause retarded growth or rickets, which can also be caused by rare genetic defects in the kidney's reabsorption of phosphate.

Toxicity

At the beginning of the twentieth century, the renowned American naturopath Dr Henry Lindlahr (1862–1924) wrote:

> *"Excess phosphorus and the acid from it overstimulate the brain and the nervous system, causing nervousness, irritability, hysteria, and the different forms of mania."*

Whether or not this view is accepted today, it is true that excess phosphorus over calcium in the first days of life can cause muscle spasms in infants.

Toxicity, called hyperphosphatemia, is rare because the body regulates any excess, and it is only usually a problem if calcium intakes are low. But too much phosphorus from supplements or in the diet can lead to an increase in blood phosphate, which may be symptomless, but it can lead to calcium deposits and hardening of soft tissues, such as the kidneys, which in turn disrupts calcium metabolism. It can therefore be a risk factor for reduced bone mass and osteoporosis. High intake of processed foods, which are often high in phosphorus, can adversely affect bone health.

Phosphorus (P)

RDA in the UK = 550 mg/day
Toxicity level = 4.5g/day

	mg/100g
1. Baking powder	8430
2. Wheat bran and dried yeast	1200
3. Yeast extract	950
4. Whitebait	860
5. Nuts, seeds, soya beans (average)	680
6. Cocoa powder and tea (average)	650
7. Sardines, cod roe and cheese (average)	500
8. Pearl barley, rye flour, self-raising flour (average)	400
9. Beans, peas, lentils, instant coffee	350
10. Muesli	280

Potassium

Potassium is present in all body cells. It has a complementary action to sodium in cell function, and levels are closely controlled by the body. Cellular "pumps" utilising sodium and potassium enable substances to move in and out of cells. Potassium is found primarily inside cells with sodium outside. Any excess potassium is excreted by the kidneys.

Potassium boosts energy and strength, and it enables nerves and muscles to function properly. It is also involved in the regulation of blood sugar levels, and is essential to the normal functioning of the heart. Eating a diet rich in potassium helps the body to get rid of excess sodium, which in turn helps to prevent or reduce high blood pressure.

"Primitive" diets, consisting of unprocessed foods predominantly of vegetable origin, supply the body with more potassium than sodium. A number of diseases seen in modern societies may be partially caused by diets containing more sodium than potassium as processed foods and meat contain more sodium than potassium while fresh fruits and vegetables contain more potassium than sodium.

Deficiency

Too much sodium in the diet—in the form of salt—may reduce potassium levels in the body. Potassium deficiency can also be caused by malabsorption, chronic diarrhoea and other gastrointestinal disorders, diabetes, diuretics, steroids, aspirin, purgatives, and laxatives.

Features of deficiency include a variety of symptoms, such as poor appetite, tiredness, depression, constipation, palpitations, muscle weakness, cramps, irregular heartbeat, and in severe cases, heart failure.

Toxicity

Potassium overload can result from excessive potassium supplements, and it is also caused by severe dehydration and kidney or adrenal failure.

Symptoms of potassium overload are stomach pain, nausea, and diarrhoea. High blood levels of potassium are very toxic and lead to rapid heart failure.

Older people may be at more risk of harm from potassium overload because their kidneys can be less able to filter out potassium from the blood, so they should not take potassium supplements without consulting their health practitioner.

Potassium (K)

RDA in the UK = 3550 mg/day
Toxicity level = 18g/day

		mg/100g
1.	Yeast extract	2100
2.	Dried apricots	1880
3.	Soya flour	1660
4.	Cocoa powder	1500
5.	Butterbeans	1160
6.	Parsley	1080
7.	Nuts (average)	750
8.	Greens (average) and garlic	650
9.	Potato, mushrooms, garlic, celeriac	570
10.	Banana, avocado, cauliflower, beetroot	400

Sodium and chlorine

In nature, sodium and chlorine are usually found bound together into salt, a condiment long treasured for its flavour-enhancing properties. Salt is essential for life and saltiness is one of the basic human tastes. It is also an excellent food preservative used since ancient times for salting, pickling, and brining to keep foods from going off and be able to store them for the lean seasons. There is evidence of salt processing of food going back to 6000 BC, and the word "salad" comes from the ancient Roman practice of salting leaf vegetables.

It is found as crystalline rock salt or dissolved in, and extracted from, seawater, and it was once an important currency, transported overseas and along salt roads. The old saying "being worth your salt" came from the habit of using salt as a payment, and the word "salary" derives from the Latin word for salt. Its value and scarcity are illustrated by nations going to war over it and using it to raise tax revenues.

Salt has also long been held in high esteem in religion and culture as an auspicious and cleansing remedy to clear an area of harmful or negative energies, and the practice of offering salt and water as invocations is thought to be the origin of "holy water" in Christianity.

And yet, only a small percentage of manufactured salt is used in food! Most of it is used in agriculture, water treatment, chemical production, de-icing, and manufacturing of caustic soda and chlorine, soaps and glycerine, the production of aluminium, and synthetic rubber, the firing of pottery, and the dyeing of textiles.

In human physiology, sodium and chloride are, together with potassium, important factors in maintaining water balance in the body, and sodium is also essential for nerve and muscle function.

Sodium chloride is found in all body fluids, in blood plasma and lymph, in the interstitial fluid found in spaces between cells, delivering materials to the cells, providing intercellular communication, and removal of metabolic waste. The interstitial fluid is made of water, amino acids, sugars, fatty acids, co-enzymes, hormones, neurotransmitters, cellular products, and salt.

Chlorine is the major element that balances sodium and potassium levels in cells. Salt requirements are closely related to water intake. Too little salt causes muscle cramps, but salt intake may have to be restricted in kidney disease or in cases of marked water retention. Infants are very sensitive to high salt intakes, especially in infant milk formulae. It is important not to give salty foods to infants since this may result in serious salt/water imbalance.

High blood pressure has been linked to habitually high salt intake. About 10% of the population have a genetic predisposition to develop high blood pressure when taking more than 3–5 grams of salt per day. An increased potassium intake minimises the effects of sodium on blood pressure.

The current average adult intake is 8 grams per day, and this is far in excess of need. In Britain, adults need less than 3 grams of sodium per day, but more during exertion—especially in hot weather—because of the loss in sweat. In high temperatures, the body conserves salt by decreasing the salt concentration in sweat, but hard manual work in hot environments, vigorous exercise, and sauna baths may all cause excessive sweating over a short period of time and may thus result in sodium deficiency. Excessive sweating, burns, severe vomiting, diarrhoea, diuretic therapy, and kidney damage can all cause loss of salt and water from the body. This leads to dehydration accompanied by nausea, dizziness, vomiting, muscle cramps, apathy, and exhaustion. Unless treated by the replacement of water and salt, dehydration may lead to life-threatening shock and circulatory failure.

The basic human salt requirement can be gained from the salt present naturally in food, but most people consume an extra 5 grams of added salt per day. Sodium chloride is added to many prepared foods and processed foods. Sodium nitrate is used as a preservative in meats. Sodium bicarbonate (baking powder) and monosodium glutamate (flavour enhancer) are also dietary sources of sodium.

In affluent societies, excess salt causes health problems. As the amount of salt needed is only a fraction of the amount routinely eaten, high blood pressure and heart disease are clear consequences.

Vegetables have a low sodium and high potassium content, and the easiest way to reduce salt intake is to eat a diet based on fresh fruits and vegetables, and to cut down on fast foods, processed meats and snacks. Since much of the salt we eat is incorporated into food, it is more effective to change what we eat rather than to reduce our consumption of table salt.

Sodium chloride (NaCl)

RDA in the UK > 6g/day
Toxicity level < 10g/day

		mg/100g
1.	Soya sauce	5493
2.	Yeast extract	4500
3.	Anchovies	3930
4.	Seaweed	2500
5.	Olives	2250
6.	Bacon	1960
7.	Smoked salmon	1880
8.	Salami	1850
9.	Prawns	1580
10.	Cheese	1410

Sulphur

Sulphur (S) is incorporated in two amino acids, methionine and cystine, and two B-vitamins, thiamine and biotin. Sulphur also forms part of skin, cartilage, and connective tissue. Its role in the body is not clearly understood but it is present in all living tissues, and it is one of the most abundant minerals in the human body.

It has antibacterial effects and is part of the group of antibiotics called "sulfonamides", although some sulfonamides have no antibacterial effect but are used as anticonvulsants (sulbutiamine), antidiabetic drugs, herbicides, and thiazide diuretics.

Sulphur is also used externally to treat skin conditions such as acne, seborrheic dermatitis, dandruff, and scabies.

Sulphur in water gives a distinct rotten egg smell—because rotten eggs contain sulphur gas! Bathing in hot springs containing sulphur and other minerals is known as balneotherapy and has been used since ancient times as an effective form of medical treatment for a wide variety of health problems.

The best dietary source of sulphur is protein-rich foods.

There is no RDA for sulphur.

Trace elements

There are ten essential trace elements:

Iron
Zinc
Fluoride
Selenium
Copper
Chromium
Cobalt
Iodine
Manganese
Molybdenum

Knowledge of the roles and requirements of the trace elements is incomplete partly because the utilisation of one trace element may be affected by the amounts of other elements present and partly because dietary deficiencies of many are unknown. The importance of some of the trace elements has only been recognised relatively recently.

They are classified into two groups: essential and non-essential, and the term "trace element" refers to any chemical element that is present in the human body in very small amounts, usually less than 0.1% by volume.

They are important for metabolism, as catalysts for enzymes, and in the transport of oxygen. The amounts required for health and the amounts that will produce a toxic effect are little different. All trace elements are toxic if consumed at higher than needed levels for long enough.

Some trace elements, including vanadium, nickel, tin, lithium, and a few other very rare substances have not yet been proven to be of vital importance for the body even though they are undoubtedly present and appear to have some influence on cell processes.

Other trace elements, including aluminium, cadmium, mercury, arsenic, and lead, do not seem to be essential for human health but are often consumed as contaminants in food or water.

Iron

Iron is an essential trace element. It plays a number of vital roles, and the body contains iron in red blood cells, muscles, enzymes, and liver stores. It is used for transporting oxygen around the body, for hormone production, for releasing energy from food, and in the elimination of toxins and waste products. Too much iron, on the other hand, is extremely toxic to cells and tissues because it can also produce free radicals—like an iron bar or a car can rust. The rust is made of free radicals. So iron levels are tightly regulated in the body to avoid both deficiency and overload.

Healthy adults contain about 3–4 grams of iron, more than half in the form of haemoglobin. It is also found in myoglobin (in muscles) and in the liver. This is why meat and liver are high in iron. The amount of iron in milk is small, so infants use their accumulated body stores to maintain iron levels during the first six months of life.

The amount of iron in the body is controlled almost entirely by the amount absorbed because losses occur only when blood or other cells are lost from the body. Menstruating women, therefore, need more iron than everyone else. Iron is also lost daily from the body via faeces and urine, but those losses are small. When red blood cells end their life, after about 120 days of service, the iron from them is not lost but recycled.

Haemoglobin is all-important as the carrier of oxygen from the lungs into the tissues of the body. Combustion is impossible without oxygen, and digestion is like a slow combustion engine. Without combustion there can be no heat production nor any elimination of waste products. It has also been discovered that iron moving rapidly in a salty solution (sodium chloride in the blood) is involved in producing electric and magnetic currents that influence cell processes. Thus iron must be regarded as one of the most important positive energy-producing elements in the body.

Absorption

Only between 5 and 15% of dietary iron is normally absorbed. Absorption is greatest in childhood and tends to be reduced in later years. It is increased when needs are greatest—for example, during periods of growth, blood loss, or pregnancy. During pregnancy, the increased need is counterbalanced by the lack of menstruation and the mobilisation of some of the mother's stores.

Iron exists in food in two forms—haem and non-haem. Animal-based foods contain haem iron, which is easier to absorb. Plant-based foods contain non-haem iron, in addition to other nutrients, which increase iron absorption.

Haem iron is absorbed unchanged while non-haem iron must be reduced to the ferrous form before it can be absorbed. Vitamin C is involved in this reaction and increases absorption significantly. Many plant foods that are high in iron are also high in vitamin C, parsley being a good example. Ancient Greeks used to crown their victors with parsley garlands, and "to need parsley" was an expression of weakness. Its reputation as a remedy for anaemia can be traced back thousands of years.

But, whatever the iron content of the diet, absorption rates change according to whether body stores are depleted or full.

The presence of phytate in a meal can also decrease iron absorption, but it is important to acknowledge that it does not block it completely. Several studies have found that even large amounts of phytate and fibre in the diet do not cause iron deficiency.

The use of cast iron posts and pans also contributes to dietary intake, as does iron-rich drinking water. I lived in the Pyrenees for a number of years where we drank spring water coming out of the iron-rich mountains, and we also used cast iron pans. I had been vegan for many years and, when I became pregnant, the local obstetrician was very surprised to find that my blood iron levels were very high, and I was far from anaemic!

Factors that enhance iron uptake are vitamin C, fructose, citric acid, lysine, histidine, cysteine, and methionine. Fruit is the best food to aid iron absorption. High altitude enhances the production of red blood cells, and haemolysis, haemorrhage, androgens, cobalt salts, low iron stores, and idiopathic haemochromatosis (a genetic defect) also encourage iron absorption.

Examples of factors that inhibit iron uptake are oxalic acid in spinach, rhubarb, and strawberries; tannins in tea; carbonate in fizzy drinks; phosphate in phytates; and excess of other metal ions, such as calcium, cobalt, copper, zinc, cadmium, manganese, and lead.

High iron stores, infection, inflammation, and lack of stomach acid also inhibit iron absorption.

Deficiency

Worldwide, iron deficiency is a common consequence of malnutrition. It is estimated that 2 billion people in the world suffer from anaemia. In developed countries, blood loss or inhibited absorption caused, for example, by excessive intake of tea, cow's milk, or calcium supplements, are more likely causes.

The National Diet and Nutrition Survey suggests that around 45% of teenage females and 30% of young women in the UK lack iron in their diet, and around 10% of them suffer from anaemia.

Causes include:	Blood loss from	– menstruation
		– gastric or duodenal ulcers
		– haemorrhoids
		– adverse effects of drugs (such as aspirin and anti-arthritic drugs that cause gastric bleeding)
		– tumours in the gastrointestinal tract
		– operations
		– excess alcohol intake
	Intestinal worms and parasites	
	Pregnancy	
	Breastfeeding	
	Low levels of vitamin C and copper in the diet.	

There is a relationship between iron levels in the body cells and resistance to disease. Anaemia leads to decreased white blood cell production and lowered immunity, and it can be the cause of breathlessness, palpitations, dizziness, persistent tiredness, mood changes, and poor concentration. In young children, iron deficiency may also be associated with depressed growth and impaired mental performance.

Toxicity

Iron overload, usually the result of taking supplements, causes stomach pain and constipation, and the cure is to stop taking the supplements. Up to 20% of people taking supplements may suffer some gastrointestinal disturbance.

Frequent iron injections, blood transfusions, various blood and liver disorders, and the hereditary disease haemochromatosis, can also produce toxic overload, ultimately leading to congestive heart failure, arrhythmia, loss of libido, arthritic joint problems, type 2 diabetes, pancreatic and liver damage. In these cases, the most effective treatment is regular removal of excess body iron by phlebotomy (drawing blood from a vein).

Ferritin is a blood protein that contains iron and it is an indicator for how much iron your body stores. Higher than normal levels can be a sign of your body storing too much iron (as in haemochromatosis or frequent blood transfusions), and it can also be a sign of liver disease, hyperthyroidism, cancer, rheumatoid arthritis, and other inflammatory conditions.

Iron (Fe) top ten (milligrams per 100 grams of food)

RDA in the UK = 9 mg/day for men and postmenopausal women
15 mg for menstruating women
Toxicity level = 20 mg/kg of body weight in one dose

		mg/100g
1.	Thyme	123.6
2.	Jellyear mushrooms	56.1
3.	Parsley, basil, oregano, bay leaf	41.5
4.	Cockles	28.0
5.	Bran Flakes	24.3
6.	Seaweed (average)	15.0
7.	Wheat bran	12.9
8.	Liver (average)	11.3
9.	Sesame, pumpkin seeds, fresh mint, treacle	10.4
10.	Beans, chickpeas, lentils, wheat germ	8.3

Note: greens such as endive, green peas and beans, Swiss chard, vine leaves, watercress, mustard leaves, and curly kale contain between 2 and 3 mg of iron per 100g; and beef, lamb, pork, and chicken contain between 1 and 2 mg per 100g. Offal, such as heart, kidney, liver, and black pudding have a higher content, between 3.6 and 20 mg per 100g.

Zinc

Therapeutically, zinc is used to treat skin complaints, prostate problems, schizophrenia, hyperactivity in children, and high blood fat levels.

Zinc is involved in several enzyme systems, and it is also necessary for normal protein synthesis and carbohydrate metabolism. It forms part of the structure of cell membranes and helps to promote the healing of wounds.

It is a constituent of insulin and prostatic secretions, and is necessary for metabolism of alcohol, for the elimination of lactic acid from working muscles, and for the efficient transport of carbon dioxide in the blood. It also helps to transport vitamin A to the skin. About 60% of total body zinc is found in skeletal muscle and 30% in bone.

Zinc is essential for growth, blood fat regulation, and protein, carbohydrate and alcohol metabolism. It promotes the elimination of waste from working muscles and insulin and seminal fluid production. It also protects against prostate disease and mental disturbance.

Zinc is present in a wide variety of foods, particularly in association with protein, although abundance or lack of zinc in the soil influences the zinc content of plants.

In a typical UK diet, about 30% is absorbed, although up to 50% can be absorbed if there is very little zinc in the diet. Absorption also increases during pregnancy, so no additional intake is necessary. Vitamin B6 increases zinc absorption significantly. Excessive zinc can decrease absorption of copper, iron, calcium, lead, and cadmium because they all compete for binding sites.

The concentration of zinc in pancreatic juice is high but is reabsorbed so losses of zinc are generally low.

Polyphosphates, which are added to many processed foods, particularly frozen and canned meats and fowl, can combine with zinc to form insoluble and therefore unavailable zinc phosphates. EDTA (ethylene-diaminetetra-acetate), used in food processing, immobilises zinc into stable insoluble chelates. Human studies have shown that large doses of calcium may decrease intestinal absorption of zinc. There is controversy over whether the fibre and phytate found in plant foods affect the body's ability to absorb zinc.

Zinc is excreted mainly via pancreatic juice into the gut but is also lost in urine and sweat. Alcohol increases urinary excretion of zinc.

Deficiency

This was first noticed in the 1958 by Dr Ananda S. Prasad, who evaluated a patient living in the Nile Delta of Egypt. The patient suffered from severe iron deficiency, but Dr Prasad noticed that he appeared much younger than his chronological age with severely stunted growth, without having reached puberty. The young man also had an enlarged liver and ate clay. Several more cases were reported. Treatment with zinc as a supplement and in the diet gave positive results, and zinc deficiency has since become much better understood, although there are still many unanswered nutritional questions regarding assessment of zinc status.

Today, it is thought that most people can get all the zinc they need from eating a varied and balanced diet, but health problems such as sudden weight loss, alcohol abuse, gastrointestinal disorders, burns, and surgery cause zinc deficiency, and a typical fast-food diet—high in fat and refined carbohydrate—is low in zinc. Porphyria, thiazide diuretics, liver disease, and kidney disease also increase zinc excretion in the urine and may lead to zinc deficiency.

Clinical features of zinc deficiency include loss of appetite, failure to grow, skin changes, impaired immunity and wound healing, loss of sense of taste and smell, skin lesions resembling eczema, especially around mouth, eyes, nose, and vagina, hair loss, diarrhoea, mental apathy, defects in reproductive organs, decreased growth rate, slow mental development, fatigue, post-natal depression, white spots on nails, and "pica" (eating dirt by children).

In the male, the prostate gland contains more zinc than any other organ, and prostate problems may respond to increased zinc intake.

Zinc is associated with the skeleton and is thought to play a major role in the metabolism of connective tissue. It is also involved in bone mineralisation and is therefore fundamental to building and maintaining bone structure.

Toxicity

Too much zinc, usually from supplements, causes nausea and vomiting, stomach pain, diarrhoea, and fever. Excess zinc intake may interfere with copper, iron, and calcium absorption. This can lead to anaemia and weakening of the bones.

Zinc poisoning may occur from drinking acidic beverages from zinc-galvanised containers.

Zinc (Zn) top ten (milligrams per 100 grams of food)

RDA in the UK = 9.5 mg/day for men • 7 mg for women
Toxicity level = 2g in a single dose; 25 mg/day long-term

		mg/100g
1.	Oysters	45.0
2.	Wheat germ and wheat bran	17.0
3.	Calf liver	12.0
4.	Beef	10.0
5.	Pumpkin seeds	10.0
6.	Dark chocolate	9.6
7.	Crab	7.6
8.	Peanuts	6.6
9.	Nuts and seeds, average	5.3
10.	Soya beans, lentils	4.0

Note: modern farming methods, particularly of pigs, have led to higher zinc intakes in humans, both directly from eating meat (especially liver paté) and also from the slurry used to fertilise the fields where food crops grow. The problem stems from zinc being added to animal fodder. The zinc content in soil that has had pig slurry added has risen by nearly 25% since 1998. The zinc is given to young piglets that are taken away from their mothers' several weeks before they would be weaned naturally. Their stomachs are not developed enough to eat solid foods and the piglets are given zinc to stop them having diarrhoea. Some 94% of the zinc is excreted and spread back onto the fields as slurry, and back into the food chain. Zinc is used as an alternative to antibiotics that are also used to solve the problem of frequent infections and diarrhoea in young piglets.

Fluoride

Fluoride is associated with the structure of bones and teeth. Drinking fluoridated water is a rich source of fluoride in Western society. Otherwise tea and seafood provide significant amounts. Fluoride combines with calcium to form insoluble calcium fluoride. There is concern about increasing amounts of fluorides in water and the food supply, which may be decreasing calcium absorption.

If water supplies contain more than 10 mg fluoride per litre, then "fluorosis" may affect consumers' health, causing abnormal calcification in muscles and tendons, nerve disturbances, and osteosclerosis. Fluorosis also causes mottling of teeth and weakened enamel, mainly in the upper jaw. The level of fluoride commonly added to municipal water is 1 part per million, but as little as 2 parts per million can cause dental fluorosis (mottling of the teeth).

Fluoride has been suggested as a treatment for osteoporosis, but results of various studies have been inconsistent.

Fluoride (F) top ten (micrograms per 100 grams of food)

No RDA in the UK
Safe intake = The upper limit is 0.05 mcg per kilo body weight per day for infants and young children.

		mcg/100g
1.	Black tea*	372.9
2.	Raisins	233.9
3.	Crab and shrimp	209.9
4.	Wine	153.3
5.	Grape juice	138.0
6.	Potato chips	115.0
7.	Coffee*	90.7
8.	Carbonated drinks*	80.6
9.	Oats	71.6
10.	Tap water (average)	71.2

*the amount of fluoride depends on the levels in the water used.

Selenium

Selenium is an antioxidant that boosts immunity and helps red blood cells to function properly.

Selenium forms part of an antioxidant, and blood levels of this enzyme increase with increasing selenium intake up to a certain point. Beyond this point, additional selenium has no effect on the amount of enzyme.

Levels in the blood, tissue, and urine all reflect dietary intake, and about 55% of dietary selenium is absorbed.

The amount of selenium in plants depends on how much they absorb from the soil, so the amount of selenium in food is very variable. Pollution and intensive farming have reduced soil selenium levels, and food processing methods also reduce the selenium content in food.

Selenium content in the soil varies widely within and between countries. The selenium content of animal products varies with the selenium content of the animal feed. Modern fertilisation practice and the spread of acid rain have also reduced the amount of selenium in our foods.

Deficiency

Selenium deficiency is not common but may be caused by high intake of processed and refined foods, and feeding babies on formula milks instead of breast milk.

Deficiency lowers immunity and is linked with cancer, heart disease, hypertension, angina, muscle pain, stroke, eye disease, cot death, and male infertility. Severe deficiency in young people causes degenerative heart disease.

Toxicity

Excess dietary intake is unusual but accidental overdose with supplements may cause hair loss, brittle nails, itchy skin rash, depigmentation, abnormal nails, and in severe cases, neurological disturbance and paralysis.

Children with a high intake of selenium may have a higher incidence of dental caries.

Therapeutically, selenium is used in cancer therapy, heart disease, and to strengthen the immune system.

Selenium (Se) top ten (micrograms per 100 grams of food)

RDA in the UK = 75 mcg/day for men • 60 mcg/day for women
Toxicity = more than 350 mg/day

		mcg/100g
1.	Brazil nuts	254
2.	Butter	146
3.	Smoked herring	141
4.	Lentils	103
5.	Apple cider vinegar	89
6.	Tuna	78
7.	Barley, wholemeal bread	66
8.	Swiss chard	57
9.	Oats	56
10.	Sunflower seeds	49

Copper

Copper helps produce red and white blood cells. It also triggers the release of iron to produce haemoglobin, and is therefore important for the oxygenation of all tissues. Copper is involved in blood cell formation, the immune system, bone formation, iron absorption, synoptic transmission in the central nervous system, the synthesis of melanin, and the maintenance of connective tissue.

It helps to keep red blood cells healthy and may protect against osteoporosis and arthritis. Copper is important in helping babies to grow, and in the development of brain, immune system, and bones.

Deficiency

Deficiency is uncommon but occurs in cases of malnutrition, malabsorption, and chronic diarrhoea. Zinc, cadmium, fluoride, and molybdenum supplements may inhibit absorption. Chelating agents, used to remove toxic minerals from the body, may also cause deficiency, and it may occur in hospitalised patients on intravenous feeding or kidney dialysis, in children with genetic defects (for example Menkes syndrome), in infants with anaemia, and in premature babies.

Symptoms of deficiency include anaemia, osteoporosis, water retention, nervous irritability, diarrhoea, lowered immunity, depigmentation, poor growth, and hypothyroidism.

Toxicity

Toxicity causes nausea, abdominal pain, diarrhoea, muscle pains,
abnormal mental states, and excess haemolysis. Excessive copper is also
thought to cause premature ageing of the skin, and long term it can
cause damage to the liver and kidneys.

Therapeutically, copper is used in the treatment of copper deficiency
and in the management of rheumatoid arthritis where copper bangles
can be effective. Some IUD contraceptive devices are based on copper.

Copper (Cu) top ten (milligrams per 100 grams of food)

RDA in the UK = 1.2 mg/day
Toxicity level = 10 mg/day

		mg/100g
1.	Beef liver	16.1
2.	Oysters	13.7
3.	Liver, average	5.0
4.	Brazil nuts	2.3
5.	Nuts and seeds, average	2.0
6.	Dark chocolate	1.8
7.	Shiitake mushrooms	1.2
8.	Split peas	1.2
9.	Potatoes	0.6
10.	Tofu	0.4

Note: processed foods, pesticides, and fungicides contain high levels of copper.

Chromium

Chromium is fairly widely distributed in foods and is found mainly in
the outer layers of vegetables. Whole grains contain chromium in the
bran and germ layers. All refined foods are low in or lacking chromium.

The highest concentrations of chromium in the body are in the skin,
fat, adrenal glands, brain, and muscle tissue.

Chromium is involved in the proper utilisation of glucose by the body.

A complex of chromium with niacin (B3) and 3-amino acids is called Glucose Tolerance Factor (GTF). This, together with manganese and insulin, is required for the conversion of blood sugar into energy. In some people, the ability to form GTF is diminished, and this may lead to diabetes and high cholesterol levels.

The increased consumption of processed foods in our society has decreased the average chromium intake. Furthermore, refined carbohydrates are quickly digested and rapidly increase blood sugar levels, which, ironically, requires the body to produce more insulin and GTF to deal with the blood sugar. Refined carbohydrate diets may thus contribute to the increased incidence of heart disease, diabetes, hypoglycaemia, and impaired protein metabolism.

Deficiency

Causes of deficiency include high intake of refined sugars and starches, a diet high in refined and processed foods, diabetes due to complete lack of insulin (chromium loss in urine), prolonged slimming regimes, severe malnutrition, and alcoholism.

There is no RDA for chromium, and only 0.5% to 2% of chromium from food and water is absorbed from the intestines.

Chromium (Cr) top ten (micrograms per 100 grams of food)

No RDA in the UK
Safe intake >25 mcg/day
Toxicity level = not set

		mcg/100g
1.	Brewer's yeast	112
2.	Beef	57
3.	Liver	55
4.	Wholemeal bread	42
5.	Wheat bran	38
6.	Oysters	26
7.	Potatoes	24
8.	Wheat germ	23
9.	Green pepper	19
10.	Eggs	16

Cobalt

Cobalt's most significant role in human nutrition is as a component of vitamin B12 (cobalamin), but it also has a role in the metabolism of fats, carbohydrates, and protein. Cobalt also plays some of the same roles as manganese and zinc, both of which it can replace in some biochemical reactions, and it takes part in the process of breaking down sugars into energy in the biotin-dependent Krebs cycle.

Cobalt the mineral forms part of the earth's crust, and it is found in most plants, including cabbage family members, lettuce and other greens, whole grains, dried fruit, fish, and animal-based foods.

As a supplement, it is best to take cobalt with vitamin B12.

Deficiency per se is unknown.

Toxicity

Toxicity is also rare but can lead to heart muscle disease, which may be caused by drinking too much beer out of cans containing cobalt. An increase in red blood cells, called polycythaemia, may also be caused by too much cobalt.

High intake can also cause goitre, which is an enlargement of the thyroid gland, and reduced thyroid activity, and it can increase blood sugar levels.

People who have had hip replacements, using metal-on-metal devices, can have high cobalt levels.

Symptoms of cobalt toxicity include fatigue, weakness, numbness in hands and feet, loss of vision or hearing, cognitive decline, heart muscle disease, and hypothyroidism.

Cobalt (Co) top ten (micrograms per 100 grams of food)

No RDA in the UK
Safe intake 5–8 mcg/day
Toxicity level = not set

The cobalt content in food is not well documented, but beans, liver, meat, fish, and eggs have the highest content. Smaller amounts are found in nuts, whole grains, vegetables, and fruit. It is also found as part of vitamin B12.

Iodine

Iodine is a vital component of the thyroid hormones that regulate metabolism and tissue repair, and promote growth and development. Most iodine in the body is found in the thyroid gland, and deficiency causes thyroid problems including goitre.

Iodine is not synthesised by the human body and must be supplied in the diet, or from supplements, medication, or iodinated contrast media.

The most reliable source of iodine is the sea. Fish and seaweeds are high in iodine. There is iodine in vegetables and grains—therefore also in animal foods—amounts depending on the level in the soil. Iodine is added to farm animal feed, so milk is a main source in the average English diet, together with iodised salt.

Via its role as a constituent of thyroid hormone, iodine could be said to stabilise and control nearly all biochemical reactions in the body. It is also thought to help regulate calcium and phosphorus metabolism and starch metabolism.

Radioactive iodine from nuclear disasters can cause thyroid cancer. On the other hand, proper amounts of normal dietary iodine can protect against the absorption of the radioactive iodine. Radioactive iodine salts are rapidly excreted if the thyroid has no need for iodine. Iodine is also used in medicine as a quick-working antiseptic with antimicrobial and antiviral properties.

Deficiency

Deficiency is uncommon in the richer parts of the world but is common in poorer countries causing goitre (enlarged thyroid) and thyroid underactivity. This results in weight gain, lethargy, constipation, dry skin and hair, and (sometimes) mental disturbance. This is because iodine deficiency usually causes lowered vitality, decreased basal metabolic rate, mental fatigue, impaired immunity, defective teeth, obesity, and slow development of the sexual organs.

In children, iodine deficiency may also cause retarded growth, thickening of facial features, and impaired mental development (cretinism). Iodine deficiency is one of the leading causes of preventable intellectual disability in children and information processing, fine motor skills, and visual problem-solving skills all improve with iodine repletion.

Note that enzymes containing copper and zinc facilitate the actions of thyroid hormones at the cellular level, and therefore deficiency of

these elements may be partly responsible for the lowered basal metabolic rate and other symptoms of thyroid hormone deficiency. Research
in the US, Japan, and Iceland has linked the incidence of breast cancer
to iodine deficiency.

Toxicity

A high intake of iodine causes thyroid dysfunction, and excess intake
can also cause hyperthyroidism, and some people are more sensitive
than others to iodine.

In fact, I treated a woman last year with hyperthyroidism presenting
soon after she was exposed to iodine-containing contrast media used
in a CT scan. She came to me as an alternative to taking carbimazole
or having her thyroid removed. With a mixture of thyroid hormone-
lowering plants in her diet and as a herb tea, her thyroid hormones
came back to normal.

After iodine fortification, such as iodised salt, was implemented
cases of iodine-induced hyperthyroidism have increased, mainly in
people over 40.

Iodine (I) top ten (micrograms per 100 grams of food)

RDA in the UK = 140 mcg/day
Toxicity level = 1000 mcg/day

		mg/100g
1.	Dried kombu seaweed	448,670
2.	Dried arame seaweed	84,140
3.	Dried hijiki seaweed	42,670
4.	Dried wakame seaweed	16,830
5.	Dried dulse seaweed	5,970
6.	Dried nori seaweed	1,470
7.	Cockles, mussels	140
8.	Cod, tuna, oysters, shrimp	100
9.	Kippers, eggs	63
10.	Salmon, butter, milk, cheese	31

Manganese

Manganese is vital for healthy bones. It is also involved in protein, fat, and cholesterol metabolism, preserving cell membranes and preventing heart disease, cancer, rheumatoid arthritis, diabetes, and epilepsy.

It is associated with a number of enzymes involved in energy production, bone formation, and protein metabolism. It is also involved in the metabolism of fats and in the production of cholesterol.

Manganese absorption is dependent on the concentration of manganese in the body. It is decreased by dietary calcium, zinc, phosphorus, and cobalt, and it is increased by dietary lecithin, choline, and alcohol.

Tissue levels of manganese are regulated by excretion rather than absorption.

Tea is exceptionally rich in manganese, and peas, nuts, spices, and whole cereals are also good sources. Processing and refining foods cause serious manganese loss.

Deficiency

Severe deficiency is virtually unknown, but absorption from the gut is inhibited by other minerals and trace elements as mentioned above.

Mild deficiency has been linked with cancer, myasthenia gravis, rheumatoid arthritis, diabetes, atherosclerosis, heart disease, epilepsy, and schizophrenia.

Manganese deficiency causes abnormal bone and cartilage formation and intervertebral disc degeneration. Other features include impaired glucose intolerance, birth defects, growth retardation, reduced fertility, reduced brain function, and inner ear problems.

Toxicity

Excess manganese—from taking supplements or in drinking water—may cause psychosis and a neurological condition resembling Parkinson's disease.

Taking high doses over a long period of time may cause muscle pain, nerve damage, fatigue, and depression.

There are no standards set for manganese but safe intakes for children are >16 mcg/kilo/day, and for adults >1.4 mg per day.

Manganese (Mn) top ten (micrograms per 100 grams of food)

NO RDA in the UK
Safe intake = 1–10 mcg/day

		mcg/100g
1.	Dried sage	25.0
2.	Wheat germ	12.3
3.	Wheat bran	9.0
4.	Pine nuts	7.9
5.	Macadamia, hazel, pecan nuts	5.2
6.	Oyster mushrooms	3.6
7.	Walnuts	3.4
8.	Muesli, chickpeas, soya beans	2.6
9.	Peanuts, coconut, almonds, sunflower/sesame seeds	2.0
10.	Blackberries, lentils, tempeh, tofu	1.3

Molybdenum

Molybdenum is an essential element in most organisms. It is a key component of three oxidative enzymes in the body. They are responsible for fat and purine metabolism and help with repairing and making genetic material.

It is found in a wide variety of foods, especially in the aerial parts of plants (the parts above ground).

You should be able to get all the molybdenum you need from a healthy diet. The best food sources are beans and whole grains.

Deficiency

Molybdenum deficiency is linked to eating refined foods. It has been associated with cancer of the oesophagus, as seen in areas of China and Iran that have low soil concentrations of molybdenum.

Deficiency can also cause tooth decay as molybdenum forms part of tooth enamel.

Toxicity

No toxic levels are set for molybdenum intake from food, but taking supplements high in molybdenum may cause joint pain. High levels of molybdenum can inhibit copper absorption and therefore cause copper deficiency.

Molybdenum (Mb) top ten (micrograms per 100 grams of food)

NO RDA in the UK
Safe intake = 50–400 mcg/day

		mcg/100g
1.	Lentils	155
2.	Beef liver	135
3.	Split peas	130
4.	Cauliflower	120
5.	Green peas	110
6.	Brewer's yeast	109
7.	Wheat germ and spinach	100
8.	Brown rice	75
9.	Garlic	70
10.	Oats	60

CHAPTER 12

Antioxidants

Antioxidants prevent cell damage by mopping up free radicals and thus preventing the oxidative chain reactions that can damage DNA. Some oxidation is normal and vital for health, as the immune system actually uses oxidative reactions to destroy microorganisms, but if the level of oxidation outstrips the body's own defensive capabilities, the resulting excess of free radicals can cause cellular damage.

Accumulated damage by free radicals is known to be an important factor in ageing and disease, and the role of antioxidants in the prevention and treatment of illness is well recognised.

Antioxidants play a preventative role in many conditions including asthma, heart disease, immunodeficiency disorders, and cancer.

PART 2

DIETETICS

U sing food as medicine is an ancient practice going back beyond Hippocrates and his famous words "Let your food be your medicine and your medicine be your food."

Like your car, your body runs better on clean fuel, and it needs an oil change from time to time to get rid of the unintended impurities that have either entered with the fuel, or that appear as a consequence of the combustion engine working.

And we are like combustion engines—every cell in the body has a metabolic system that converts fuel into energy. The miracle is that the body knows how to feed every single cell, of the 30 trillion it consists of! Each one is fed and watered, and has its rubbish collected, so that it can function in harmony with all the other cells and make it possible for us live a healthy and fulfilled life.

CHAPTER 13

Naturopathic health principles

In naturopathic terms, health is based on three basic principles:

1. The vital force within the body restores and maintains health:

The vital force is that which enables the body to heal itself. It is more than the body's ability to make antibodies against infectious disease. It is a force that allows the body to maintain health and balance in the face of a changing environment.

Life force depends on: Hereditary factors
                          Constitution
                          Acquired characteristics.

In the body, each cell is connected to its surrounding cells, and they all communicate with each other. It is your life force that keeps them alive and well. You can influence that communication by the way you live, and it is my conviction after many years of practice that all disease comes from separation and the stress it provokes.

2. Disease is an expression of the vital force working to restore health:

If an individual gets over a cold in two to three days, this shows good resistance. A cold that drags on for more than a week show that the body is finding it difficult to recover. A healthy person has greater resistance to disease and is more able to return to a balanced state of health after illness than a person who was unhealthy in the first place. This concept is at the root of the argument between Louis Pasteur (1822–1895, French chemist and microbiologist), who thought germs should be killed to prevent them invading us, and Claude Bernard (1813–1878, French physiologist), who insisted that germs are everywhere and that the trick is to be healthy and live alongside them.

Germs and pests are only doing their job, like everything else in nature. They decompose what is already decomposing into another lifeform. Worms in the soil transform decaying plant material into healthy soil containing all the nutrients from the previous plant for the new plant to grow in. We are part of nature, whether we like it or not, and our bodies are part of an ecological evolution in which the strongest genes survive and the weakest are transformed to give life to others.

Of course, some people are able to live long and, seemingly, healthy lives despite abusing their bodies with unhealthy habits, but all they are doing is taking advantage of their healthy genes supplied by their ancestors who lived long and healthy lives on natural diets in more balanced environments.

Certain illnesses may be considered helpful since they improve our general level of resistance; for example, childhood illnesses that may be necessary for the development of a good immune system. Colds, influenza, and occasional bowel disturbances can also be considered as normalising processes, as long as they do not occur too frequently or for too long.

3. An illness affects the whole person:

In assessing a person's nutritional status and diet, the following points need to be considered:

1. Previous medical history
2. Family history
3. Diet diary, recording dietary intake over a minimum of 5 consecutive days

4. A record of all supplements and medication being taken and why
5. Current nutritional needs according to occupation, hobbies, family, and stress levels
6. General information regarding state of mind, behaviour, and attitude
7. Physical assessment, weight, height, and age.

Nutritional status is gauged by the extent to which a person's physiological need for nutrients is being met in terms of wellbeing, physical and mental performance and resistance to disease. Detecting nutritional imbalance or deficiency can be difficult and requires a good knowledge of the basics (proteins, fats, carbs, vitamin, and minerals).

To obtain a healthy diet, most people would benefit from:

- Cutting total fat intake by 25%
- Cutting saturated fat intake by 50%
- Cutting extrinsic sugar by 50%
- Cutting salt by 25%
- Increasing dietary fibre by 50%

This goal could easily be reached if the whole population followed a naturopathic diet consisting of 50% raw food and plant-based foods only.
    According to the famous naturopath and scientist Henry Lindlahr (1862–1924):

> "natural food for animals and humans is that food which appeals to the senses of sight, taste, and smell in the natural condition, as it comes from nature's hand. Any food which needs disguising by cooking, spicing, and pickling is not 'natural'."

The orthodox view that the most healthy thing is to "eat what agrees with you" is not good advice to people who have become addicted to stimulants and certain other acquired tastes. In cases of food allergy, it is often found that the food a person has the greatest craving for is the thing they are most allergic to.
    It is curious to reflect that we have become accustomed to eating soured, hardened milk in the form of cheese and decaying flesh in the form of meat, and to drink fermented grapes, apples, and barley in the form of wines, ciders, and beers. We did not enjoy these tastes from birth but had to get used to them in the same way as you have

to get used to smoking before it becomes a pleasure. Likewise, people who give up eating meat and dairy products for a few months find these foods a disappointment when they taste them again and may experience unpleasant disturbances in their digestion such as nausea, digestive cramps, wind, and diarrhoea. If you stop eating nuts, fruits, or vegetables for months or years they taste no worse when you taste them again.

CHAPTER 14

Nutritional assessment

First it is necessary to assess the calorific value of a diet. Calories provide the daily energy for activity, tissue maintenance, and digestion. Tissue repair requires more energy than the simple breakdown of nutrients. Whether in the diet or from body stores, calories are obtained from either carbohydrates, proteins, or fat.

The conversion values are as follows:

1 gram of carbohydrate = 4 kcal
1 gram of protein = 4 kcal
1 gram of fat = 9 kcal

The difference in calorie density shows how smart it is to carry energy reserves as fat, since you can carry over twice as many calories per gram or kilo. This is good for birds that fly from one end of the earth to the other on their fat reserves, but it is bad for dieters since it means it takes 4½ days to lose one kilo of fat, presuming your calorie intake is zero, and your need is 2000 kcal/day.

In a healthy diet, the proportions of carbohydrate, protein, and fat should be as follows:

Carbohydrate   70% of total food intake. Of these 90% should be intrinsic carbohydrates, as opposed to extrinsic (carbs with added sugar). The NHS Eatwell Guide recommends 37% should be starchy foods, such as whole grains, potatoes, breakfast cereals, bread and pasta, the rest coming from fresh fruit and vegetables.

The current average UK starch intake is 27%.

Protein   10% of total food intake. The current average UK intake is 12%. There is no such thing as first- and second-class protein.

Fat   15–30% of total food intake. Of these, the amount of saturated fat should be less than the amount of unsaturated fat. The current average fat intake in the UK is close to 35%, 13% of which is saturated fat.

Fibre   >30g per day. The current average intake of UK adults is 20g.

CHAPTER 15

Food as medicine

Junk food is well known to have an unhealthy effect on the body, and by the same token, it is possible to use nutritious food as medicine.

There are two types of diet used in naturopathic treatment: the anabolic and the catabolic.

Anabolism is the process in which the body forms new tissue by synthesising simple compounds into more complex molecules.

Catabolism is the process in which the body breaks down nutrients and converts complex molecules into simpler ones. Production of energy is catabolic.

The body is constantly breaking down and regenerating tissues as part of normal daily life, and catabolic/anabolic diets aim to support or enhance these existing processes.

Catabolism and anabolism occur simultaneously in the body and are usually in a balanced dynamic equilibrium. At certain times in life, however, the balance may tip more towards one or the other.

During childhood, pregnancy, and convalescence, rapid tissue growth is needed, so these are anabolic phases. Disease, stress, injury, and immobility cause catabolism to predominate.

Put simply, a catabolic diet is used to detoxify and cleanse the system, and an anabolic diet is used where the individual needs building up.

The pioneering endocrinologist Hans Selye (1907–1982) believed that all illness is a manifestation of stress, and that stress is the cause of all illness. He devised the concept of the *General Adaptation Syndrome*, which states that the body has the ability to integrate all bodily systems to maintain a balanced state but, if the stress is extreme or unusual or long-lasting, the normal mechanisms may not be sufficient for the body to cope.

The general adaptation syndrome

There are three stages in the general adaptation syndrome:

1. The Alarm Phase: the most dramatic; a short, acute fight-and-flight response. This is designed to give the body instant energy to deal with any danger.
2. The Resistance Phase: this allows the body to continue fighting by breaking down carbohydrates and fats for energy. It is designed to help us deal with emotional difficulties, performing strenuous tasks, resisting infections and so on. This phase lasts longer than the alarm phase but, if it fails to deal with the problem and carries on for too long, the body enters into the third stage.
3. Exhaustion: the total collapse of the body. During this stage, the individual develops secondary infections or complications to an illness. It is the beginning of chronic disease. During the exhaustion phase, the individual's ability to promote healing is so poor that the vital force becomes weaker and weaker. Chronic responses that may develop in this stage include:

angina	depression
asthma	headaches
autoimmune diseases	irritable bowel syndrome
heart and circulatory disorders	reduced immunity
cancer	ulcerative colitis
common colds	ulcers
diabetes	

Health and nutritional assessment

During a health and nutritional assessment, the three phases of the general adaptation syndrome are used as guidelines to determine which nutritional approach is needed.

The main thing is to work out how to make a positive change today that will rekindle the vital force. The most important part of that process is to change the negative thought patterns that are connected with your illness. It doesn't matter how long it has been going on, you can start making changes today.

According to Hans Selye and many medics and healers after him, the stress factors you encounter are only part of the problem; the most important part is how you deal with them. Thoughts are things, and what we choose to think and say today will create the path we take tomorrow. As Eckhart Tolle says, "the point of power is always in the now". Overcoming disease is a journey, a healing journey, that starts with a thought and carries on with action.

First of all, it is important to make the change from victim to captain of your own ship, taking responsibility for what happened in the past and also for making positive changes that will shape the future. Although modern medical practice is combative—fighting disease—the naturopathic approach is to see disease as a friend that is telling us to change. The modern medical model suppresses the body's efforts with medication and treatment protocols that drive away symptoms and combat disease. The naturopathic approach rekindles the inherent life force and assists nature's healing potential by increasing health, and thus creating an environment that heals the person on all levels. Disease is a cleansing process bring about change for the better. In fact, naturopaths consider that many acute diseases are what naturopaths call "healing crises" by which natural forces cleanse and heal, and as a way to rest and repair and become stronger.

The naturopathic way of supporting this process is to encourage elimination of accumulated toxins and waste products by supporting natural processes. This restores a natural environment for healing and creates or recreates healthier habits, thereby supporting the life force in its work. Last but not least, naturopathy nourishes the blood with natural constituents that assist the body in creating a healthy environment that is the basis for any healing journey. Remember, a healthy bloodstream is important because it is the blood that carries nutrients to and takes away waste from every single one of the 30 trillion cells the human body consists of. This is why old herbals always talk about "blood cleansers".

CHAPTER 16

What is a healthy diet?

This is a good question the answer to which keeps changing. It has changed many times during the years I have been in practice. On the other hand, the same principles as Hippocrates held to still stand and, from a naturopathic viewpoint, a healthy diet consists of foods that support the person's many different needs without putting an extra load on the body.

In practice, this means eating plant-based foods as close to their natural state as possible, and limiting foods that are manmade as much as possible.

If a diet is varied, it is not difficult to cover all nutritional needs, and supplements are only needed in times of imbalance.

Eating for health

Eating for health means to become free from addictions—to caffeine, alcohol, sugar, fat, meat, and dairy—and enjoying natural foods instead. It is not difficult in itself, but it can be hard because there are many other reasons to eat apart from to simply nourish the body.

The simplest way to eat for health is to base your diet on plants and eat all foods as close to their natural state as possible. The more refined and processed a food is, the more likely it is to be unbalanced in terms of macro- and micronutrients. Take potatoes, for example: when they are boiled or baked, they can provide a perfect balance of nutrients and keep whole nations supplied with energy, but when processed into chips or crisps, they contribute to the combination of obesity and undernourishment that is so common today.

When you eat foods that only supply calories, but little in the way of nutrients, it is easy to overeat because your body will feel undernourished and lacking in the micronutrients it needs to feed cells and tissues. The other problem is that when carbs are easily available, they cause spikes in blood sugar that are quickly followed by the release of insulin to transport the sugar into the tissues where it is stored. That means a drop in blood sugar, which is most easily replenished by eating and absorbing more sugar, rather than getting it back out from storage. So, the body craves more sugar, and the vicious circle continues.

If, on the other hand, you eat plant-based foods as close to their original state as possible, your body does the processing during digestion, and therefore the calories are less easily available and take longer to be absorbed. As they are broken down, the micronutrients they contain are in a slow, steady stream that enhances absorption.

There may be times and places where meat and dairy are necessary for survival, but the idea that our ancestors based their diet on meat is absurd. It may come from archaeologists finding bones near palaeolithic camps—but that only bears witness to the slow degradation of bones, not to the variety of plant foods that have long decomposed. If you think about it, the energy needed to hunt and catch, slaughter and cut up and cook an animal is considerable, and it would be strange if prehistoric people hadn't discovered the edible roots, leaves, flowers, grains, seeds, nuts, and fruits. We know that they used plants as medicine too.

A true paleo diet would be plant-based with very little meat and dairy. If you consider what foods are most easily available in most parts of the world, it is clearly green leaves. And when the leaves fall, the energy of the plant withdraws into the roots, which are the perfect winter food. But before they fall, the plant sets seeds in the form of grains, nuts, seeds, and fruits. These are what the plant wants us to eat, so we can help spread seeds and sow new plants. Fruits are full of sugars made from the sun, and if dried they will keep all winter. Nuts and seeds are laborious to harvest and prepare, but they are highly nutritious so also very valuable to collect before the winter.

The fats and oils we get from nuts and seeds are almost impossible to extract if you have to do it yourself. They are also very high in calories (9 kcal per gram), so should be used sparingly.

Observations of hunter-gatherers still living in the wild in Africa, where the men hunt and the women gather, have measured that the calorific expenditure from hunting is equal to the gain, leading to the conclusion that the tribe actually depend on and live from the plant foods gathered by the women.

But most of us no longer live in the wild! We have food shops and supermarkets to hunt and gather in. Next time you go to a supermarket, have a look around at how much of the food you see is in its natural state and how much is manmade. Only a small percentage is unprocessed.

In naturopathy, the simplest way to eat a healthy diet is to concentrate completely on unprocessed foods. If you do, you will find that many of your ailments disappear by themselves because you take a load off the body and give it better conditions to heal itself when it is freed from the unnatural nutritional challenges food processing adds.

Food, as we find it in nature, contains nutrients, water, and waste. The waste is the indigestible portion of the food, such as fibre, the vital role of which is clear as we learn more about the importance of the gut biome.

Symbiosis vs antibiosis

There is no waste in nature! Everything is about collaboration and symbiosis. We knew that once, and people living in the wild still know it. It is only civilised nations that have forgotten and thus favour competition and antibiosis or antagonism. This is also known as amensalism, where a non-symbiotic, asymmetrical interaction between two species in which one is harmed or killed by the other, and one is unaffected by the other. The term amensalism is often used to describe strongly asymmetrical competitive interactions.

Parasitism is a close relationship between species, in which one organism, the parasite, lives off the host, causing it harm. The entomologist E.O. Wilson (1929–2021) has characterised parasites as "predators that eat prey in units of less than one". The human race is a planetary parasite.

Predation is defined as an organism killing and eating other organisms. Scavengers, parasites, and herbivores are all predators if they kill their prey, but there are ways of being a scavenger, parasite, or herbivore that does not kill the target. Scavengers prey on organisms that are already dead and thus make use of their energy instead of the dead body causing pollution. Parasites can live in a mutually beneficial relationship with their prey, by keeping it alive. Herbivores that only eat part of the plant live in a symbiotic relationship with the plant world because they help them spread their seeds, and they also supply useful fertiliser for the plant to grow and breathe out carbon dioxide for the plant to breathe in and thus produce oxygen and carbohydrates during photosynthesis.

Plants are the basis for all animal life on earth because they convert solar energy into chemical energy that we can use to grow and live active lives. Whether you choose to pass energy through another animal before you eat it is another matter. But there is no doubt that the best you can do for your own health and for the survival of the human race is to eat plants and refrain from killing.

A healthy diet should be composed mainly of fresh fruits and vegetables because they are high in micronutrients and low in calories. Concentrated protein, fat, and carbohydrate foods should be eaten sparingly. The detrimental effects of excess carbs, fats, and proteins do not show up as long as the body is able to make use of and eliminate them, but once that capacity is diminished, problems start.

The ketogenic diet

The worst case of varicose veins I have come across in practice was in an otherwise healthy man in his thirties who had followed a ketogenic, high-fat/low-carb diet over a number of years. The ketogenic diet replaced fasting as a treatment for epilepsy, and it makes sense that eating more fat might help to correct nerve conduction anomalies in the brain. It has been successful in children, but it is not without side effects, although the side effects may be milder than the ones produced by epilepsy medication. Common side effects include constipation, acidosis, and low blood sugar, raised blood fat and cholesterol levels; supplements are necessary to counter the dietary deficiency of many micronutrients. Long-term side effects include stunted growth, bone fractures, kidney stones, and dyslipidaemia (an abnormal amount of lipid in the blood), which is a risk factor for coronary artery disease, stroke, and varicose veins…

Eat less

In naturopathic terms, a healthy diet not only involves what and how much to eat but also when. The simplest guide is to only eat when you are hungry, while remembering that hunger and appetite are two very different things. An appetite can be aroused by smelling food or seeing others eat, but it disappears again if it isn't followed, like a habit or an addiction.

If you eat as your hunger dictates, and you are sure it is hunger, not craving, you will find yourself healthier, more energetic, and in tune.

Eat less by eating slowly and chewing your food well. Chewing releases digestive juices and ensures better absorption. The famous naturopath Bernarr Macfadden (1868–1955) said, "Chew your food! Your stomach has no teeth!", and Virgil MacMickle (1897–1967) added, "Taste your food! Your stomach has no taste buds!"

These naturopathic pioneers treated myriad people and diseases using these simple principles of following a healthy diet. Of course, it is also true that "one man's meat is another man's poison", and different diet regimes are called for at different times and in different situations. Where you live, how you are, what you do, how old you are, what time of year it is—all influence how much food you need, and what sort.

When animals are unwell, they stop eating, and the same is usually true for humans; the return of the desire to eat after illness is usually taken as a sign of healing. A catabolic diet allows for the energy normally used for digesting food to be applied to the process of getting well, and it helps the body to focus on repair and rejuvenation. After a catabolic diet the body is able to absorb nutrients from food more effectively and to deal more efficiently with waste materials. It is a bit like having an oil change in your car. Everything runs more smoothly afterwards.

A catabolic diet regime is suitable for treating illness and as a detox. It can also be used as a slimming regime, as it uses your stored fat reserves to create energy. Since most waste and toxins are accumulated in your fat, it is usually a great relief to get rid of it.

On the other hand, there are times in life when an anabolic diet is what you need, a wholefood diet designed to increase vitality and provide the strength necessary to recover from chronic illness. It can be used in all circumstances where catabolic dieting would be too challenging, when resources are low and vitality is weakened. It can be a first step back to health if you feel you have tried everything to cure your health problem but without success.

Anabolic diets often include particular foods and herbs for their specific medicinal actions, and also for their high content of vitamins, minerals, enzymes, and immune-stimulating constituents. They create circumstances that make it easy for you to get well.

CHAPTER 17

Diets and dieting

The American National Weight Control Registry (NWCR)—a national database of individuals who have achieved successful weight loss—contains information on over 10,000 Americans over the age of 18 who have managed to maintain a 30 lb (13.5 kg) weight loss for a year or more. About 45% of those participating lost weigh on their own, while 55% had participated in formal weight-loss programmes; 20% had used low-calorie liquid diets; 4.3% had used weight-loss medications; and 1.3% had undergone gastric bypass surgery. Almost all had previously tried several weight-loss methods without success. Of those who were successful, 61% followed a more rigorous diet than before, and 81% exercised more. The average successful slimmer expended about 2800 kcal per week on exercise (about one hour a day). This evidence confirms that diet without exercise and lifestyle changes rarely produces lasting weight loss, and suggests that structured programmes make the process of dieting more effective.

As most people wishing to lose weight also want to improve their long-term health, it is vital that slimming regimes incorporate the principles of healthy eating. Good nutrition is now accepted worldwide as the most powerful and cost-effective way of enhancing health and vitality, and of avoiding serious illness in the long term. A well-nourished body is better able to support and sustain weight loss.

Getting the most out of your slimming diet

Whatever type of slimming programme you choose, there are a number of nutritional and lifestyle guidelines that will help to ensure that your diet is as healthy and effective as possible:

- **Eat a balanced wholefood diet:** from a nutritional perspective, the best diet consists entirely of unprocessed foods. It should be high in unrefined complex carbohydrates (60–65%), fibre, and simple fruit sugars, and contain no refined sugar at all. It should provide a moderate amount of protein (10–15%), a controlled amount of unsaturated fat (20–30%), and very little saturated fat.
- **Eat fresh fruits and vegetables:** the easiest way to improve your diet is to greatly increase your fruit and vegetable intake and cut out dairy products altogether. There are plenty of plant-based alternatives on the market including soya, rice, oat, and almond milks, nut butters, plant-based cheeses, and pure vegetable margarines.
- **Eat more fibre:** soluble and insoluble fibres are crucial for slimming because they are low in calories and yet give a feeling of fullness. They also improve fat and cholesterol metabolism, and aid digestion.
- **Eat proper meals:** to achieve weight loss it is better to eat proper meals than snacks. If you need to snack, eat natural wholefoods, such as carrot or celery sticks, apples, oranges, bananas, papaya, pineapple, nuts, seeds, or wholemeal sugar-free biscuits.

Catabolic diets

Catabolic diets involve fasting and controlled diets of varying stringency to cleanse and promote healing.

Catabolic diets are beneficial in the alarm or resistance phases of the general adaptation syndrome since, during these phases, the individual's vital force is still strong. The duration of a catabolic diet varies according to individual need.

Catabolic diets promote cleansing and rejuvenation because they allow the body to break down and burn old and diseased tissues and, at the same time, to release stored toxins for elimination.

Since the average diet often contains empty calories and toxins in the form of hormones, antibiotics, pesticides and herbicides, preservatives and colorants, it is not easy for the body to keep the tissues "clean". Autoimmune diseases and allergies may be triggered by a slow but constant ingestion of substances that compromise the body's natural functions and balance.

In daily life, the body deals with ingested toxins by "walling them off" in safe storage spaces such as fat and bone. During a catabolic diet, the body is using up stores and therefore eliminating toxins that may have built up over a long time. It does not break down tissues indiscriminately but decomposes and burns diseased, damaged, old and dead cells and tissues preferentially. Blood sugar and protein levels are normal while the burden of digestion is removed. The eliminatory organs—lungs, kidneys, liver, and skin—work more efficiently. Because of increased elimination, the individual may feel nauseated and have headaches. The urine may become dark and perhaps smelly, and the breath offensive. Skin eruptions, excessive sweating, and catarrhal mucus production are common accompaniments.

The digestive system as a whole is given a rest, and, on completion of a catabolic diet, absorption of nutrients and food transit time are greatly improved. All physiological, nervous and mental functions are stabilised and rejuvenated.

Catabolic diets are graded according to severity:

1. Raw fruit and cooked/raw vegetables with rice
2. Raw fruit and cooked/raw vegetables
3. Raw fruit and vegetables
4. Mixed fruit—this includes a mixture of fruits according to preference and objective.
5. Mono-fruit—one variety of fruit or vegetable is eaten. Normal meal times are kept but only one type of fruit or vegetable is consumed.
6. Fasting—the most eliminative and effective. In a true fast, only spring/mineral water is allowed. In a less stringent fast, fruit juice, and alkaline vegetable juices are allowed. All juices are diluted with 50% water. The individual can drink as much as they like but a minimum of 8 large

glasses (2 litres) should be drunk per day. Tea, coffee, alcohol, and fizzy drinks should be avoided as they burden the system chemically.

When a diet of this nature is prescribed, it is important to instruct the individual in how to prepare for it (see below), to prepare them for "healing crisis symptoms" such as headache, nausea, dizziness, dark smelly urine, and bad breath. It is also important to return to normal again slowly, introducing one food at a time, with stimulants, meat, and dairy added last, if at all. Note that the end of a fast is a good time to detect food allergies.

Fasting

Animals withdraw from eating when they are unwell. Restrictive diets and abstinence from food have been used as a form of treatment for various disease for many centuries. For example, in pharaonic Egypt fasting was used as a treatment for syphilis and gonorrhoea.

Fasting rejuvenates and detoxifies the system. It allows the body to heal itself. It is used primarily in the treatment of acute disease, but also has a place in the management of chronic complaints such as asthma, arthritis, stomach ulcers, allergies, high blood pressure, heart disease, colitis, enlarged prostate, and kidney disease.

It is important to be aware of the effects of fasting and of the "healing crisis" (see later). It is also important that a person fasting is relaxed and in a suitable environment.

If a fast is to continue for more than three days, a slow introduction and a gradual return to normal eating is necessary. During a long fast it is important to be in contact with a suitably qualified practitioner who can monitor your wellbeing closely.

Aims

There are two main aims of fasting:

1. To give the body a rest: the process of digesting, absorbing, and metabolising food requires a lot of energy. During a fast, this energy is saved and can be channelled into healing processes.
2. To allow the body to concentrate on elimination. The body's energy can be used to remove waste products and toxins.

In other words, the body is allowed to have a spring-clean with no new substances added to the system. In this respect, the body can be visualised as your mailbox where post is sorted into useful mail and junk mail. If there is a lot of incoming mail and it contains a lot of junk mail, sooner or later your mailbox overflows and it becomes impossible to keep up.

Similarly, a person who over-eats and whose diet contains a lot of non-nutritious junk food is pushing their body towards an unbalanced, diseased state. Provided the situation is not too advanced, a fast (stopping the incoming mail) will allow the system to clear the back log.

The idea is to rest the whole body, so your energy is focused on repair of the body.

Points to consider before fasting

1. Preparation	Psychological and mental preparation involving considering your reasons for fasting and what is likely to happen. A transition diet is advisable.
2. Rest	Plan your fast, and start at a time that ensures you can get as much rest as needed, in a restful environment.
3. Activity	Conserve energy, but move, walk, enjoy the sunshine. You can carry on working during a fast, as long as you pace yourself.
4. Warmth	Don't get cold! Since you haven't got the warmth from your internal combustion engine while fasting, you will feel colder. It is important to keep warm because eating your fat reserves does not generate the same heat as you get from the usual digestive processes.
5. Water	Drink as your thirst dictates. Drink little and often but at least 2 litres of water per day. The water should be as pure as possible.
6. Breathing	Every body cell needs oxygen, so if you can't go to a pure-air mountain resort, do breathing exercises and get as much fresh air as possible where you are.

7. Sunshine	Traditionally, lying in the sun 8 minutes per day was prescribed for fasting patients at health spas.
8. Suffering	It is never as bad as people think! The first two to three days on water are the hardest while your metabolism gets used to the idea of using your fat reserves instead of getting ready meals. But remember—birds fly hundreds or thousands of miles on their fat reserves. It can be done!
9. Contraindications	If you suffer from anorexia, advanced heart disease, advanced cancer, diabetes, or tuberculosis, or if you are pregnant or breastfeeding, fasting is not for you. Having said that, in early pregnancy, morning sickness may improve after a brief fast.

Effects of fasting

During this bodily spring-clean, all the eliminative and excretory organs are stimulated. Hence the urine may become darker and possibly begin to smell more during the first days. After 1–2 weeks the urine becomes clear again and loses its strong odour.

The breath may smell and the tongue can become coated. You can scrape off the coating with a teaspoon or a tongue-scraper. The tongue clears from the tip backwards until the mouth and tongue are clear and the breath is fresh—unless you get dehydrated, then it starts to have an unmistakable sickly-sweet ketosis smell.

Initially, you may sweat more and your bowels may become looser. If you fast on water, you will stop having bowel movements, and it is advisable to take an enema after a week or so to clear out any faeces left behind.

Weight loss varies from 250 grams per day to 1.5 kilos per day, with an average of ½ to 1 kilo per day, most in the beginning where you lose both fat and water, and before your body becomes more economical with its calorie use.

Some people feel weak in the beginning as the body operates on less calories. A return to vigour is an indication that the body has freed itself of toxins.

Over the years, I have had many fasting people in my care, and sometimes the results are remarkable:

A young woman in her mid-twenties who suffered from severe period pain went on a water fast, and after a couple of weeks had a period out of the normal rhythm, and passed what looked like an old lifeless encapsulated embryo that must have been lodged in her uterus for several years. Her period pains and menstrual problems were completely gone after the fast.

A man in his thirties with digestive problems, and difficulty with digesting fat, went on a water fast. After ten days on water, he had a bowel movement. Nothing came out apart from several gallstones. He could hear them drop and wondered what it was! His digestion was fine when he started eating again, and he could eat fat without any problem.

A woman in her fifties, also with digestive problems, and who had travelled in Asia and South America, had a bowel moment after a week on a water fast, and passed a huge parasitic worm!

These are only a few examples of the powerful effects of fasting.

The lean season

Fasting is also a good way to become aware of why we eat and who is in charge of our food choices. In former times, when we didn't have supermarkets and food shops to keep us supplied, people living off the land would often experience scarcity towards the end of winter and the beginning of spring.

Carnival traditionally marks the beginning of Lent. The origin of the word can be traced back to the Latin expression *Carne Levare* or *carnelevarium* meaning 'farewell to the flesh'. This was a traditional ritual where the spirits of winter were driven out to make way for summer and fertility, a rite of passage from darkness to light, and an opportunity to eat well before stocks ran out.

Together with the spiritual aspect, the Carnival ritual involved the practical side of consuming the remaining winter stores of meat, butter, and lard before they started to decay. Meat for the winter was slaughtered in November, so by February it was getting past its sell-by date and had to be eaten. Before Lent began, all animal food and drink were consumed in a giant celebration involving the whole community.

During Lent, no parties or celebrations were held, and people abstained from eating rich foods such as meat, dairy, fat, and sugar.

As with many other Christian festivals, Lent is based on these much older traditions. After the Carnival, people said goodbye not only to eating of flesh but also the desires of the flesh, with a huge frivolous party held behind masks, with permission to experience wild abandon and hilarity, perhaps to make sure most wild desires were lived out before the time of betterment.

Carnival falls on the Sunday before or on Mardi Gras (Fat Tuesday), also known as Shrove Tuesday or Pancake Day, the last day before commencing the fast and the religious obligations associated with Lent, which begin the next day, on Ash Wednesday. Shrove Tuesday is the day of confession and self-examination, of considering what wrongs need to be repented, and what amendments to life or areas of spiritual growth need dealing with.

Lent begins on Ash Wednesday, the first day of fasting, and lasts for 40 days until Easter, reflecting the 40 days Jesus spent fasting in the desert. The name Lent is derived from the practice of burning the palm branches blessed on the previous year's Palm Sunday, and marking a cross of the ashes on the forehead of worshippers.

In all the various versions of Lent, the tradition is to abstain from eating rich foods containing meat, dairy, eggs, and sugar. Apart from simplifying one's diet during Lent, it is also a time to abstain from partying and for making an effort to repent for sins and become a better person, for example by letting go of a bad habit; or doing something that reinforces a spiritual connection; or by giving time and/or money to charity.

Whether you call it Lent or spring detox, it is a good time for cleansing and rejuvenation, spiritual as well as practical. In nature, the early spring is the time where everything starts to reawaken, and the energy takes an outward direction again. Green sprouts and flowers suddenly appear, the light grows stronger, and so does our need for renewal. It is time for new life and new beginnings. Nature serves many free detoxifying foods at this time of year—green shoots filled to the brim with vitamins, minerals, antioxidants, and other phytonutrients—to renew and recharge our batteries and free us from the grip of winter.

In religious terms, the aim of fasting period is, "through prayer and abstinence", to conquer evil in the world as well as in body, mind, and spirit, and from the earliest times it has been a time of cleansing and detoxification. By abstaining from the normal amount of calories, the body has a chance to use up the fat reserves that have been gathered through the winter, which is a good idea as the body also has a habit of storing waste and toxins in its fat deposits.

At this time there is a natural urge to go on a diet and get rid of the winter fat, have a good clear-out in house and garden, as well as body and mind, getting ready for the return of the summer sun.

Fasting guidelines

There is an old proverb that says getting out of the door is 90% of the journey, so if you have already decided to try a spring-cleanse, the sooner you start the better.

Digesting, absorbing, and metabolising food uses a considerable amount of energy, and restricting your food intake during a period of healing allows some of this energy to be channeled into the process of healing. Gently cutting down on the food you take in helps the body to dispose of stored-up toxins and allows the organs responsible for getting rid of waste products (kidneys, liver, skin, and lungs) to work more efficiently. A simple diet consisting of fresh fruits and vegetables encourages your natural self-cleaning ability.

A detox-fast consists of a series of simple steps. You take one at a time and you can decide to remain at each step or go further as you wish. In principle, you can decide to remain at each level for as long as you wish, and your fat reserves allow. And remember, it is a time to be good to yourself and your body, by giving yourself time to rest and regenerate.

For each step, drink plenty of pure water and weak herb teas. The return to normal eating should also be done very carefully, and you should spend as many days gently going back up the steps and returning to a normal diet as you spent going the other way.

Start by cutting out stimulants (coffee, tea, green tea, chocolate, alcohol), sugar, and all foods containing these.

Move on to also avoiding meat, fish, shellfish, dairy, bread, nuts and seeds, pulses, vegetables, and fruit, one step at a time. See how far you can go.

Take your time, see how each step feels and enjoy what you eat. Don't spend too much time thinking about what you don't eat. This is an easy temptation to become obsessed with. Explain to yourself that this is only a short period of time, which makes you healthier, more energised and happier with yourself. It does!

Your goal is to do this detox diet over 40 days, but how stringent you make it depends entirely on how you feel. Try to make time for yourself in this period. Rest as much as you can and make sure you get out in the fresh air each day. Go for as long a walk as you can manage.

Eat organic! And eat as much as you like of your chosen foods. Drink pure water whenever you are thirsty, and remember—when we feel we want to eat something, it is because we are thirsty!

Fruits and vegetables contain a lot of water and are easily digested. They have a high vitamin and antioxidant content, and they are a good laxative.

Here's an overview of a traditional spring detox. Go only as far as you feel comfortable with but challenge yourself too. For many people, the first step is the hardest—coming off the stimulants often causes a headache for a couple of days.

Step 1: Cut out all sugar, alcohol, and stimulants (including caffeine from tea, coffee, and chocolate).

Step 2: Also cut out all meat and fish, and animal fats.

Step 3: Also cut out all dairy products, and products containing dairy derivatives.

Step 4: Also cut out all grains. Eat only nuts and seeds, beans and pulses, raw fruit and cooked/raw vegetables.

Step 5: Also cut out all nuts and seeds. Eat only beans and pulses, raw fruit and cooked/raw vegetables.

Step 6: Also cut out all beans and pulses. Eat only raw fruit and cooked/raw vegetables.

Step 7: Also cut out all vegetables. Eat only fruit. Remember some vegetables are also fruits—including avocado, tomato, cucumber, peppers, aubergine, pumpkin, courgette, and squash.

Step 8: Also cut out all fruit. Drink only water, diluted juices and gentle herb teas.

During the detox, it is interesting to reflect on who is in charge of your life.

Is it your desires? Is it your habits? Your addictions? Your cravings? Your emotions? Your fears? Your ambitions? Your feelings of guilt or inadequacy? Your material needs? Is it your family? Your friends? Your partner? Your job? Your boss? Your bank? Your beliefs? Your dreams? Or is it yourself?

This is the time to get in touch with your self and find out what a wonderful being you are and have always been. Eating sunshine, which is what you literally do when you stick to fresh fruit and vegetables, makes it easier to get in touch with the spiritual aspects of yourself. People talk about being on a 'detox high' where it becomes clear what really matters. Take this chance to get in tune.

Detox herbs

Nettle

One of the important detox foods is stinging nettle (*Urtica dioica*) one of the world's most misunderstood weeds. Eat it during the first seven steps of a fast or detox, and drink it as a tea when you get to the eighth step.

Despite nettle's reputation, it is both delicious and nourishing as a vegetable, and the 'sting' disappears with cooking or blending. It is also a useful natural medicine, which has been used for centuries in spring cures as a 'blood cleansing' remedy. Nettle is nutrient-rich with a high content of vitamins A, C, K, B1, B2, B3, and B5, as well as calcium, magnesium, iron, potassium, bromium, selenium, silica, zinc, serotonin, chlorophyll, lycopene, and omega-3 and -5 fatty acids.

In the old herbal traditions, nettle was seen as a warming and drying remedy able to drive out cold and damp conditions, and to give the body energy. Nettle's modern use as circulatory stimulant and diuretic reflects this old understanding, and its ability to detox the body and clear out accumulated waste and toxins makes it extremely useful for treating arthritis.

In immunodeficiency, chronic debilitating conditions, and cancer, the nettle has a unique ability to revive and replenish, improving the body's ability to deal with difficult circumstances as well as deliver many of the building blocks that are needed for health and wellbeing. The nettle is a mild but effective diuretic, freeing the body from excess fluid and at the same time strengthening blood vessel walls. Its considerable iron content also makes nettle useful for anaemia.

Spring is the best time to start using nettles in food and drinks, but if you decide to create a nettle patch in your garden—keep on picking from the same patch—you will have fresh young nettles all summer and well into winter. Only the young shoots are used. If you pick them regularly from the same plants, you can keep on picking fresh shoots almost all year. Pick them—wearing gloves—wash them and simmer them in a little water for about 5 minutes. Remove from the water with a slotted spoon, chop them finely and use them, together with the cooking water, in soups, stews, and sauces. They can also be used like spinach.

Nettle tea

per cup
2 fresh young nettle shoots, or 1 tsp dried
1 inch pieces of fresh ginger, finely sliced
1 thick slice of organic lemon or lime
1 cup of boiling water

Place the nettle, ginger and lemon in a cup or a teapot, add the water and infuse for 5–10 minutes. Adding the fresh ginger makes the tea especially warming, as ginger is a "diffuse stimulant", directing the circulation to the extremities.

Feeling cold is a side effect of fasting, caused by having no food to metabolise but eating your fat reserves instead. So, keep warm!

Cleavers

Cleavers (*Galium aparine*) is another excellent herb for detox. It can be used safely for many different health problems, and the reason it is helpful for detox is that it is a brilliant tonic to the lymphatic system. It is also a soothing diuretic that helps rid the body of metabolic waste and toxins.

Cleavers contains flavonoids, glycosides, coumarins, caffeic, salicylic, gallotanic, and citric acid. It has a long history of medicinal use as an alterative, anti-inflammatory, gentle diuretic, astringent, antitumour, skin healing, and fever-lowering remedy.

It is one of the first plants to appear in spring, growing abundantly in hedges, wasteland and woodland gardens, enjoying dappled shade but growing almost anywhere. The young shoots and leaves are used.

Cleavers recipes

Cleavers tea: a small handful of fresh sprigs, or 1–2 tsp dried, to a cup of boiling water. Infuse for 15 minutes. Drink 3–4 cups per day. Goes well with nettle.

Or add a long sprig of cleavers to a bottle of water and make a cold infusion. It is delicious and tastes a bit like cucumber.

You can also juice the fresh plant and take 1 tablespoon at a time.

To make a cleavers smoothie: blend a handful of fresh cleavers with fruit, vegetables, and ice.

Elimination diets

If you suspect you have a food intolerance, but you are unsure what you are intolerant to, one way to find out is to keep a diet diary:

Carry a notebook with you everywhere each day for a week and record EVERYTHING you eat and drink and the time you had it. You need to write things down at the time as it is easy to forget afterwards!

At the end of each day, write down how, and where, you've been that day, whether you've had any allergy symptoms, such as migraine, sneezing, or stomach ache. If you are suffering from arthritis, you should also note whether your arthritis was better or worse, on a scale of 1–10, that day. Food allergy symptoms can start up to 24 hours after the allergen was consumed, so keeping a diet diary enables you to look back and identify possible offenders more easily.

If after a week it is clear that you have good days and bad days according to what you eat, you can start to create your own personal elimination diet by keeping your diet diary up to date and eliminating the foods you have found are not good for you.

Healing crisis

A healing crisis, although perhaps not always particularly pleasant, is a positive sign we look for in naturopathy—by crisis we mean turning point, and the healing part of the concept speaks for itself.

The healing crisis often occurs naturally as an acute illness where a fever makes you lose your appetite and makes you rest so the energy normally used for digestion and action can be used for healing. Digestion is one of the most energy-consuming activities, so directing that into healing has a remarkable effect.

The elimination that happens during times of fasting and rest is remarkable. All the eliminatory organs spring into action. Mild depression, irritability, insomnia, weakness, teeth feeling coated, skin rash, aches and pains, bad taste in the mouth, headache, and diarrhoea are common symptoms of a healing crisis. The blood pressure may increase slightly on the third day but should then return to normal.

All these are good signs! They show that the body's clean-up operation is under way. People react in different ways, however, and if you are doing a long fast you should have a practitioner monitor your wellbeing.

Ketosis is also a sign of a healing crisis. It refers to any elevation of blood ketones and is a metabolic state that happens when the body burns fat instead of glucose for energy. It produces a particular "acetone breath"—which usually implies dehydration. The more serious ketoacidosis is a metabolic state caused by uncontrolled production of ketone bodies. The most common cause is diabetes, but it can also be caused by alcohol, drugs, toxins and, rarely, starvation in the presence of an additional metabolic stress factor. Ketoacidosis needs medical attention.

The intensity of a healing crisis depends on how much accumulated waste you are carrying. The body continually weighs up conflicting demands and calculates risks for long-term survival. It will sacrifice the least essential tissues in order to conserve and protect the vital ones.

It is healthy to allow the body to have a regular healing crisis by removing internal and external obstacles for this to happen without force, letting the body follow its own instinctive healing process. This is done by removing all the habits that have contributed to the unhealthy condition.

A properly managed acute disease or fast once or twice a year does wonders for the overall health of the body, mind, and spirit. Never being ill or taking time off to detox is not necessarily a sign of health. It may also be a sign of the immune system being suppressed by stress.

The features of the healing crisis also include going back through the diseases you have previously suffered from as the body returns to interrupted tasks of healing problems that were suppressed.

The duration and intensity of the healing crisis is very variable and individual. The more vital power you possess the shorter and stronger the reaction. This is why children can become acutely ill and then suddenly completely well again. Generally, the older you are, the weaker the reaction, and you will find that emotional and psychological problems may also rear their head, wanting to be processed and released.

In summary, the healing crisis is like a detox, a time when your earthly vehicle is cleaned from top to bottom, the entire system upset and short-tempered, and normal life interrupted. The process may happen without deliberate provocation, in the shape of an acute disease, usually after a period of stress; or it may be deliberately provoked by imitating the state of acute disease.

A healing crisis is not something to fear or try to avoid; it should be welcomed as a sign of vitality and be allowed to run its course. To quote the famous naturopath C. Leslie Thomson (1914–1992): "It is literally a rejuvenating process, and an encouraging experience."

Convalescence

Do you know the feeling after an acute illness where you wake up with the fever gone, feeling much better, longing to get out and get on with your life again? Then you get up, go out, and realise that while you felt fine lying down, that is not the case when you start moving and are exposed to different temperatures and environmental challenges. If you persevere, it may cause a backlash and the illness returns with increased vigour.

That principle applies to all illness, and also to detox and fasting. Although this is not recognised in modern medicine, the old tradition of taking time to rest after a period of repair is vitally important for long-term health.

During the healing phase of any illness, there is always a susceptibility to further illness, because there is less vital energy available. For this reason, it is extremely important that the period of healing is followed by a period of convalescence, during which energy is restored. Even minor illness or detox deserve a period of convalescence to allow time for the healing process to be completed. Sadly, many people return to work at the first opportunity after illness, and though this may cause no obvious problems for some months or years, if the pattern continues a sense of deep tiredness or exhaustion starts to become a major feature of daily life. At this point, a period of rest and relaxation is vitally necessary to restore inner balance. Without it, chronic illness of some sort will develop.

A few extra days back at work are not worth the possible months or years of chronic illness that can result when simple illness is repeatedly not allowed proper time to heal.

However, convalescence doesn't mean staying in bed. Gentle exercise, time spent in the fresh air or enjoying a non-strenuous hobby can all help the process of true recovery.

Anabolic diets

If you are suffering from a chronic illness, or have been through a period of physical, mental, emotional, or spiritual stress, a gentle healing diet is beneficial to provide resources for healing. It is made up of organic foods that are highly nutritious, easily digested, and easily absorbed and used by the body to regain health and wellness.

The diet contains the right amount of protein for growth and repair, and plenty of complex carbohydrates for sustained energy. It is low in fat but contains all the necessary essential fatty acids, and it is high in vitamins, minerals, and other healing phytonutrients.

Meat is not suitable for a gentle healing diet because it is a very concentrated food, containing no fibre, usually high in saturated fat, and it may contain residues of growth and stress hormones, antibiotics, nitrates, and other additives or harmful substances, depending on how the animal it came from was treated.

Good sources of complex carbohydrates include gluten-free grains such as quinoa, amaranth, oats, and rice; and also roots and tubers such as parsnips, celeriac, carrots, potatoes, sweet potatoes, yams, and beetroot.

Good sources of protein include beans, peas, and green leaves.

Organically grown vegetables, either raw or cooked, boiled, baked, or steamed, depending on your taste, your state of health, and your digestion, are at the core of the anabolic diet because of their high content of vitamins, minerals, and phytochemicals.

Start with cooked vegetables if you find raw foods hard to digest and add some raw ones little by little.

Eat one or two pieces of fruit each day, but in this diet the aim is to build up resources by eating food that provides steady energy without too many short bursts upsetting blood sugar levels. Most fruits contain simple sugars (fructose) that are digested and absorbed into the bloodstream more quickly than the complex carbohydrates (polysaccharides) in vegetables. Choose fruits that improve digestion, such as papaya, pineapple, banana, and grapefruit. Lemons are high in vitamin C and low in sugar.

Nuts, seeds, and olives all contain unsaturated and omega fats that are good for health.

Drink only water—at least 5 glasses per day, and herb tea, but avoid the artificially flavoured ones.

Foods to avoid:

- All sugars and foods containing added sugar
- All refined or processed foods and fast foods
- Fruit juices
- Stimulants, such as black/green/white tea, coffee, alcohol, chocolate, fizzy drinks
- Non-prescription drugs and supplements
- All foods containing saturated fats
- Additives
- Dairy products
- Meat
- Fish and shellfish.

If you suffer from an arthritic condition, you should also consider excluding tomatoes, peppers, aubergine, acidic fruits, spinach, rhubarb, strawberries, and vinegar.

Menu suggestion:

- Start the day with a glass of hot or cold water with lemon juice.
- Breakfast: gluten-free, sugar-free muesli with fresh berries and almond milk.
- Lunch: vegetable soup and salad.
- Supper: vegetable stew with beans or lentils, rice and greens.

Alkalising foods

The idea of eating an alkaline diet, also known as an acid–alkaline diet or alkaline ash diet, is that what you eat can alter the acidity or alkalinity (pH value) of your body.

In fact, a complex interplay between various body systems ensures that the pH of the blood is always maintained at a constant level between 7.35 and 7.45. In other words, the blood is always mildly alkaline.

The idea behind eating an 'alkaline diet' is that the foods you eat either make it easier or harder for your body to maintain the blood at a constant pH level. The suggestion is that 'acidic' foods create an internal environment that promotes disease, whereas 'alkalising' foods promote health. By choosing foods described as alkalising, you certainly can improve your health. Such foods support good bone health and help you to maintain a lean body. They can also lower the risk of having high cholesterol, high blood pressure, stroke, dementia, and kidney stones, and help reduce pain and inflammation. There is also some evidence that an 'alkaline diet' may help prevent the development of cancer, and possibly improve the efficacy of chemotherapy, as well as reduce the effects of stress on the immune system.

"Acid-forming" foods include meat, fish, dairy, eggs, grains, coffee, black tea, sugar, artificial sweeteners, high-sodium foods, peanuts, and alcohol.

"Alkalising" foods include vegetables, legumes, fruits, and nuts.

CHAPTER 18

Medicinal plant foods

Using food as medicine is not only about nutrients and treatments, it is also about getting to know the medicinal value of common foods so you can use them deliberately to improve health and treat disease.

Here is a small selection of the thousands of medicinal plants in the world. I have chosen plants that I believe you will be familiar with, and that are easy to get from your greengrocer, garden, or hedgerow.

Avocado

The avocado pear originates from Central America. It was an important component of the diet of the native Aztec people but was little known to the rest of the world until the early twentieth century. Avocados are now popular all over the world and grown commercially in many tropical and subtropical regions.

The avocado grows on an evergreen tree *(Persea americana)*, a member of the bay leaf family (Lauraceae), and is also known as alligator pear and butter fruit. The tree starts producing fruit when it is three years old, and a healthy avocado tree can continue to yield fruit for hundreds of years.

The fruits are normally picked before they are fully ripened. On average, an avocado takes about a week to ripen at room temperature. The process can be accelerated by placing it in a paper bag with an apple.

The avocado is a highly nutritious fruit that can be used to replenish vitamin and mineral loss, especially potassium. It contains more potassium than a banana as well as several other important nutrients and powerful antioxidants, including vitamin C, E, K, B-complex, magnesium, manganese, zinc, carotenoids, beta-carotene, glutathione, fibre, oleic acid, omega-3 and -6 fatty acids.

The antioxidants mop up free radicals—the destructive molecules known to trigger the development of cancer and heart disease.

The phytochemicals in avocado have strong anti-inflammatory and antifungal properties. They work by inhibiting the germination of fungal spores, and so make the avocado useful in the treatment of internal and external yeast infections.

The particular combination of nutrients and micronutrients found in the avocado stimulates the immune system, enhances antibody production and acts as a mild vasodilator, relaxing the muscles surround blood vessels, reducing blood pressure and the risk of stroke.

Eating avocado helps protect the skin from the effects of ageing and maintains hair, mucous membranes, sweat glands, nerves, muscles, and bone marrow in good condition.

Avocados differ from other fruits in being extremely high in fat—75%—most of which is monounsaturated oleic acid. There are many health benefits associated with eating a diet high in monounsaturated fat such as this. In particular, such fats reduce levels of LDL cholesterol in the blood and have a beneficial effect on the composition of blood fat in general. Monounsaturated fat also helps to stabilise blood sugar levels.

Most of the rest of the fat found in avocados is polyunsaturated. As the fruit ripens, the small amount of saturated fat it contains steadily turns into polyunsaturated fat.

Avocados also contain phytochemicals called beta-sitosterols, which reduce the absorption of cholesterol from food. Beta-sitosterols are widely used in the manufacture of blood cholesterol-lowering drugs.

Beetroot

Beetroot *(Beta vulgaris)* is a member of the amaranth family (Amaranthaceae). The root is sweet and strong-tasting when raw but has a gentler flavour when cooked. The leaves taste a bit like spinach for which they can be used as a substitute. It is native to southern Europe and is derived from the sea beet *(Beta maritima)*, which grows wild on the coasts of Europe, North Africa, and Asia.

Beetroot has been cultivated for food and medicine since the earliest times. It was so treasured by the people of ancient Greece that it was routinely offered—on a tray of pure silver—to the God Apollo in his temple at Delphi.

Beetroot is known to herbalists as the vitality plant. In the old English tradition, beetroot was said to be good for the blood, and this is reflected in its modern use in the relief of chronic illness of all sorts, including chronic infections and ME (myalgic encephalomyelitis).

The root is rich in phytosterols, saponins, protein, sugars, vitamins, and minerals, especially B6, folic acid, iron, and magnesium; and the leaves are a good source of calcium, and vitamins A and C. It has a high content of the anthocyanin pigment, betacyanin, which is a powerful antioxidant, and is also rich in fibre, which helps improve bowel function and lower blood cholesterol levels. The synergistic effect of betacyanin and fibre may explain beetroot's protective role against bowel cancer, and many practitioners have also reported encouraging results in cases of other cancers, particularly leukaemia. There is evidence that eating beetroot can cause cancer cells to either revert to normal or die, by altering the rate of cell respiration.

It is not 'a cure for cancer' but it may help extend the length and quality of life of sufferers.

Beetroot stimulates the immune system by improving cell respiration and tissue oxygenation by encouraging the production of new red blood cells. The enhanced cell respiration helps keep the heart, muscles, and nerves in good condition. It also helps stabilise the body's pH (acid–alkaline balance). This is important for immunity because bacteria thrive when the body is acidic.

Its unique mixture of minerals and phytochemicals resists infection, boosts cellular intake of oxygen, and treats disorders of the blood, liver, and immune system.

Beetroot is a cheap, non-toxic, and widely available supportive treatment for conditions involving the blood and immune system by improving cell oxygenation, and this effect may explain its reputation for increasing overall vitality. It can be used—raw, juiced, blended, boiled, stewed, or baked—as a medicine to improve vitality in all chronic illness.

Beetroot juice has been used in the treatment of hepatitis, nephritis, and polio. The Nobel Prize-winning physician and microbiologist Professor Robert Koch (1843–1910) claimed to have found it useful in the treatment of these diseases.

The average adult dose is one medium-sized root per day. The root has no harmful side effects and is well tolerated by most people. It needs to be eaten over a relatively long period of time to improve general health and vitality.

A word of caution—the red pigment in beetroot may colour faeces and urine red. This effect is harmless and disappears as soon as you stop taking the root.

The leaves contain oxalic acid, like spinach, and should not be eaten with caution by people suffering from kidney stones or arthritis.

Blood-purifying cure

Juice equal amounts of beetroot, carrot, celery, tomato, and lemon. Drink 1–2 wineglasses per day for 3 weeks.

Bilberry

Bilberry *(Vaccinium myrtillus)* is also known as "European blueberry". This lovely, sharp-tasting berry is native to the cool heaths, moors, woodlands, and mountains of Scandinavia, Europe, Asia, North America, and Canada. Like the blueberry, it is a member of the heather family (Ericaceae). The Latin name "myrtillus" refers to the leaves resembling myrtle leaves.

Records of using bilberries for medicine go back to Hildegard of Bingen (1098–1179), who recommended them to induce menstruation, and they are still used by herbalists to relieve period pain.

The dried berries can be used as an infusion to calm diarrhoea, and they have a gentle, cooling, astringent, disinfectant effect that makes them useful in reducing inflammation.

Both the berries and the leaves are used in herbal medicine. The berry contains anthocyanin flavonoids, pectin, thiamine (B1), ascorbic acid (C), beta-carotene (A), glucosides, and tannins. The active constituents act synergistically to increase the beneficial effects of bilberries on health.

During the Second World War, Royal Air Force pilots used bilberries in an effort to improve night vision during night bombing raids. Since then, studies have shown that eating bilberries does, in fact, influence adjustment to darkness and visual acuity. Further research suggests that bilberries have the ability to increase blood flow and oxygenation in the eye, making them effective in treating eye problems such as diabetic retinopathy, macular degeneration, cataracts, and glaucoma.

Their effect on microcirculation also makes them useful in the management of Raynaud's disease, and they are also used to relieve the symptoms of varicose veins and haemorrhoids.

The anthocyanins in bilberry are strong antioxidants that improve the health of connective tissue, prevent tissue damage by free radicals, and suppress histamine release, thus decreasing inflammation. Bilberries may also reduce the incidence of blood clots and atherosclerosis, and their protective effect on collagen and connective tissue helps reduce the ill effects of rheumatoid arthritis and emphysema.

Anthocyanins also decrease capillary fragility and reduce the permeability of the blood brain barriers.

Research shows that bilberries have strong antiviral properties and are able to inactivate the tick-borne encephalitis (TBE) virus.

Dose: eat 50–100 grams three times per day.

Bilberries may theoretically cause low blood pressure and low blood sugar, and there is a potential, theoretical, additive effect with anticoagulant medication.

Blueberry

The blueberry (*Vaccinium corymbosum*) is, as the name suggests, dark blue, and they have a distinctive sweet, slightly acidic taste. Native to North America, where native Americans used the whole plant for food and medicine. These days, their increasing popularity because of their therapeutic effect as well as for their great taste means that they are grown commercially all over the world, making it possible to enjoy them fresh almost all year round.

Wild blueberries grow throughout North America, Europe, and Asia. They are often mistaken for another blue berry, the bilberry (*Vaccinium myrtillus*), which is also commonly gathered and eaten in Europe. Both are members of the heather family (Ericaceae). It is easy to distinguish them from each other by cutting the berries in half: ripe blueberries have white or greenish flesh, while the flesh of bilberries is coloured purple throughout. Both prefer a slightly acidic habitat in a good compost as you would use for heathers or rhododendrons.

Blueberries are high in vitamin C, A, E, K, B-complex, potassium, manganese, copper, anthocyanins, flavonoids, mucilage, tannins, and fibre. They are a tasty, low-calorie snack, and a delicious dietary supplement.

They are called *the antioxidant super-berry* that helps protect body cells by neutralising free radicals in the bloodstream, thus reducing the risk of cancer and degenerative illness, dampening inflammation, and reducing the likelihood of contracting viral and other infections.

The anthocyanin also helps improve night vision and eyesight, as well as ease tired eyes, and relieve more serious eye problems such as cataracts, glaucoma, and macular degeneration.

Consuming blueberries or bilberries on a regular basis increases memory and learning ability, and lessens symptoms of depression. They may thus be useful in the management of Alzheimer's disease. They also help lower blood cholesterol and prevent heart disease and high blood pressure. Their tonic effect on blood vessels is also useful for treating varicose veins and haemorrhoids.

The blueberry's tonic and antibacterial abilities increase in the dried berries, which can be used as a simple and effective treatment for diarrhoea. Like cranberries, their close relative, blueberries contain a mucilage that protects the lining of the urinary tract and prevents bacteria from attaching themselves to the bladder wall, making them beneficial against cystitis and other urinary tract infections.

People with diabetes also benefit from blueberry's low glycaemic index as well as its ability to lower blood sugar. Dieters can enjoy them as a low-calorie, low-fat, high-fibre supplement to their regime as they are also thought to help burn fat and increase metabolic health.

Dose: eat 50–100 grams three times per day.

Brazil nut

This delicious South American seed is one of the richest natural sources of selenium and vitamin E. They are also high in monounsaturated and polyunsaturated omega fats.

Eating tree nuts improves cardiovascular health and lowers the risk of high blood cholesterol, heart attack, stroke, and type 2 diabetes.

Brazil nuts are also important for hormonal health because selenium is essential for hormone production, and deficiency can impair sleep, mood, concentration, and metabolism.

The thyroid gland is dependent on selenium to activate thyroid hormones by converting T4 into T3.

The powerful antioxidants have anti-ageing properties that can help guard against many disorders, including cancer, inflammation, fungal infections (such as candida), and immunodeficiency disorders.

The Brazil nut, also called the para nut, cream nut, and castanea, is the edible seed of a giant tree, *Bertholletia excelsa*, that grows in the Amazon rainforest. It is an important source of nutrition, and income, to the local population. Most Brazil nuts are collected from wild trees. They grow in clusters of 8–24 nuts enclosed in a woody, fibrous fruit capsule that looks like a cross between a coconut and a cooking pot with a lid.

Brazil nuts are extremely nutritious with high levels of protein and fibre, as well as unsaturated fat, selenium, zinc and other minerals, plus substantial quantities of vitamin E and B1. It is the combination of vitamin E, selenium, and omega oils that gives the Brazil nut its special immune-enhancing properties. These important nutrients work synergistically, each improving the performance of the other to boost immune system function.

Even a moderate increase in selenium intake is beneficial to the body's self-defence mechanism. However, it is possible to get too much of a good thing. Taking excess selenium as a food supplement can result in selenium toxicity, which can cause hair loss, dizziness, fatigue, and skin problems. Fortunately, the Brazil nut selenium package provides a natural safety limit because brazil nuts satisfy hunger before the selenium content reaches toxic levels. Many other foods of plant origin also contain selenium—the amount depending on the plant's ability to absorb it from the soil. Unfortunately, in many parts of the world, modern agricultural practices have depleted the soil of selenium, providing yet another good reason for preserving the Amazon rainforest—Brazil nuts!

Eating just one Brazil nut per day will satisfy your need for selenium, and the combination with zinc and vitamin E has been shown to be effective in treating prostate problems and preventing prostate cancer.

The recommended dose is 1–3 nuts per day.

Some people are allergic to Brazil nuts. Genetically modified soya beans may contain genes from Brazil nuts, and so may trigger an allergic reaction.

Cayenne pepper

Cayenne or chilli pepper *(Capsicum annuum/C. frutescens)* comes from a genus of flowering plants with red or green peppery fruits belonging to the nightshade family (Solanaceae). They all contain capsaicin and have a characteristic hot, sweet, fruity flavour that becomes more complex when the fruits are dried.

The hotness of chillies is measured in Scoville Units, named after Wilbur Scoville (1865–1942)—best known for his creation of the "Scoville Organoleptic Test", now standardised at the Scoville Scale. He devised the test and scale in 1912 while working on a system to measure pungency, spiciness, or heat, of different chilli peppers.

Scores on the Scoville Scale range from zero (for the sweet bell pepper) to the current official Guinness World Record holder as the world's hottest pepper—the Carolina Reaper at 2.2 million Scoville Units (SHU)!

Cayenne pepper comes from the French Guianan region of Cayenne. It is an extremely hot, long, thin, pointed, red/brown chilli with a distinctive taste, and usually dried and ground into a fine powder, often using both seeds and pods.

Cayenne is very high in vitamin A, C, E, K, and B6, carotenoids, steroidal saponins, and capsaicin, which is the main active constituent. It stimulates circulation, especially towards the mucosa in the digestive tract, promoting blood flow and increasing vascular permeability.

Cayenne is one of the purest of all stimulants and one of the most effective diaphoretics. It stimulates the heart and circulation, and increases blood flow to the tissues, producing natural warmth and increasing metabolism. It strengthens the heart, arteries, capillaries, and nerves, and helps increase peripheral circulation to warm up cold hands and feet.

It is also antioxidant with anti-inflammatory properties, and it can be used as a natural antiseptic, digestive stimulant, and food preservative. Recent research indicates that cayenne may provoke endorphin release in the brain, creating a sense of pleasure and wellbeing, and it can be used as a natural painkiller, systemically as well as topically. It is also used to relieve the pain associated with shingles *(Herpes zoster)*, joint pain, and headaches.

Capsaicin may help lower blood cholesterol, and it is used to increase the blood supply to the digestive organs, indicated in gastric and digestive insufficiency, enhancing processing abilities of the digestive organs and easing colic, wind, and indigestion. It is contraindicated in ulceration and inflammation of the digestive tract.

Dose: very individual, but 100–500 mg per day is a good guideline.

Hot chillies should be handled with care—wash your hands well after touching them, and make sure you avoid contact with your eyes and other sensitive parts of the body. Removing the seeds will reduce the hotness.

Cayenne is a natural anticoagulant and should be avoided when taking anticoagulant medication. Cayenne can also irritate stomach ulcers, and should not be used by breastfeeding mothers.

Cherry

The cherry tree *(Prunus avium* and *P. cerasus)* is a member of the rose family (Rosaceae), and it takes three to four years to start bearing fruit. All the fruits ripen simultaneously on the tree, so local sweet cherries are only available for a very short season; on the other hand, they are easy to freeze and use later, and they are also grown commercially all over the world, so they are in season somewhere all year round. The more sun they get, the sweeter the taste and, as they prefer cool winters and hot sun, cherries are well suited for growing in mountains.

They contain vitamin C (14% RDA), B1, B5, B6, folate, potassium and magnesium, malic acid, pectin, fibre, and sugars. They also have a high content of melatonin and antioxidants, including anthocyanin, melanin, lutein, carotenoids, phenols, and quercetin.

The anthocyanins in cherries have been shown to be powerful anti-inflammatories, able to reduce the pain from arthritis, fibromyalgia, and injuries, and also lowering the uric acid content of the blood, making them a traditional remedy for gout.

Cherries also boost energy and are beneficial to the heart, muscles, and nerves. They reduce platelet stickiness and can help prevent blood clots.

Eating cherries or drinking cherry juice can help improve your natural sleep cycle and be a good remedy for insomnia. Melatonin is a natural hormone produced by plants, animals, and people. It plays a key role in regulating the internal body clock. Melatonin also helps maintain optimum brain power and may help slow the development of age-related chronic diseases like Alzheimer's. The combination of melatonin and anthocyanins makes cherries an excellent brain food.

Curly kale

Curly kale *(Brassica oleracea acephala)* is a member of the brassica family (Brassicaceae), which includes cabbage, broccoli, and Brussels sprouts. They are all packed with vitamins, minerals, and phytochemicals that guard against bacterial and viral infection, heart disease, and cancer.

Curly kale is also known as "borecole" from the Dutch word *boerenkool*, meaning "peasants' cabbage". It is derived from wild cabbage *(Brassica oleracea)*, which is native to southwestern Europe and the Mediterranean region and grows on seaside cliffs. Opinions differ over when the wild cabbage was first cultivated—estimates range from a few hundred to thousands of years ago—but it has been developed into a number of edible varieties.

Although the edible brassicas originated in temperate zones, they are now cultivated all over the world, and a common characteristic is that they hold a lot of water in their leaves, making them fleshy and succulent foods. Like other members of the family, curly kale stores large amounts of nutrients in its leaves.

Curly kale is an invaluable winter vegetable with an extremely high content of vitamins A, C, and K, as well as minerals and protective phytochemicals. It is also one of the tastiest of the cabbage family and easily overwinters, even in cold winters, to provide important nutrients when little else is growing.

Its active constituents combine to facilitate oxygen transport to the tissues, support immunity, aid liver function, and play a part in controlling blood fat and cholesterol levels. It also helps the body to release and use the energy in food.

Curly kale contains three important groups of protective phytochemicals: glucosinolates, flavonoids, and sterols. Glucosinolates protect against carcinogens, and also help reduce the activity of oestrogen in the body, and therefore have a dual role in protecting against oestrogen-related cancers. Flavonoids stimulate the immune system. They chelate (combine with) metals and make blood platelets less sticky, thus protecting against abnormal blood clotting and preventing heart disease. Sterols influence the absorption of cholesterol from food and its metabolism in the body. They also affect the production of steroid hormones.

Curly kale thus promotes the health of the heart, nerves, and muscles, and protects against high blood pressure, cardiovascular disease, and autoimmune diseases. It is also good for the skin, encourages wound healing, and the maintenance of healthy cell membranes. It may also protect against oestrogen-sensitive cancers.

Because of its vitamin K content, curly kale encourages normal blood clotting, and it also helps regulate protein and fat metabolism and improve iron absorption, facilitating the production of haemoglobin and red blood cells.

Dandelion

Dandelion (*Taraxacum officinalis*) is a member of the daisy family (Asteraceae). The name comes from the French *dente-de-lion*—teeth of the lion—and is a reference to the characteristic saw-tooth shape of the leaves. The Latin name *Taraxacum* comes from the Greek words for disorder *(tarax)* and remedy *(akos)*. Dandelion is also called *pis-en-lis* in French, referring to the leaves being strongly diuretic, potentially causing you to wet your bed if you drink it in the evening!

Since medieval times, dandelion has been widely used as a spring tonic and blood cleanser with a particular affinity for the liver and kidneys.

It is a bitter and astringent plant with a high content of bitter principles, natural plant steroids, phenolic acids, flavonoids, mucilage, inulin, pectin, carotenoids (vitamin A), vitamin C, iron, magnesium, zinc, and potassium. The potassium content is very beneficial in a diuretic remedy, as diuretics can cause potassium depletion.

Dandelion leaves are an excellent source of vitamins and minerals. They are strongly diuretic and so can be used to relieve water retention caused by heart disease, for example, and useful for high blood pressure. They are also anti-inflammatory, nutritive, and bitter.

The root is a general tonic, with particular actions on the liver and kidneys. It stimulates the digestive system, especially the liver, and is useful in any condition of liver and/or gallbladder inflammation and stasis. It is also a gentle laxative, and it helps the body to eliminate toxic waste, so has a traditional use in the treatment of eczema. The plant steroids inhibit cold sores (*Herpes simplex* virus) and glandular fever

(Epstein-Barr virus), and recent studies have also shown a powerful inhibitory effect on mammary tumours.

Dandelion tea is a traditional spring-cleaning remedy made by pouring boiling water onto the leaves and leaving them to infuse for 5–10 minutes. Drink in the morning!

A dandelion broth to improve liver function is made by simmering the sliced root in water (1 tsp per cup) for 15 minutes, straining and drinking 1–2 cups per day.

The roots can also be roasted to make dandelion coffee.

Both leaves and roots are delicious in stir-fries, and the leaves are excellent in salads and sandwiches, or prepared like spinach and used as a side dish.

Use dandelion with caution in case of gastritis or digestive inflammation or ulcers, and in case of gallstones or kidney problems. It may interact with antacids and have an additive effect on diuretics, anticoagulants, diabetic medication, steroids, and potassium supplements.

Dandelion is very easy to grow and popular with wildlife. Small birds love the seeds.

Elderflowers and elderberries

The elder (*Sambucus nigra*) has a long history of use as food and medicine, and in the household. The generic name *Sambucus* may be an adaptation of the ancient Greek word *Sambuca* and refer to an ancient musical instrument. Native Americans called it "the tree of music" and used the young stems to make pipes and whistles. Mature elder wood is hard and light, excellent for whittling and carving tools and utensils. It contains a soft pith that is easily removed, leaving a hollow tube to blow in. This was also used as bellows to get a fire going, and the old Anglo-Saxon word for fire, *Æld*, may be where the name "elder" comes from.

Elderflowers contain antioxidants, mucilage, sterols, pectin, tannin, and volatile oils. They are anticatarrhal, anti-inflammatory, expectorant, circulatory and immune-stimulant. The combined effect of the active constituents is to enhance natural resistance, and to promote perspiration—removing heat from the body, and cooling fevers—so they are excellent for viral infections, especially respiratory tract problems such as colds and flu, as well as hay fever and other allergic symptoms, and catarrh.

Cold elderflower infusion soaked in clean pads and placed over the eyes can also be used to relieve eye strain and inflammation.

The berries have a high content of fibre, and they are rich in vitamin C, A, and iron. They also contain vitamin B-complex, potassium, and calcium, together with antioxidants and tannins. They were once a staple ingredient in many North American and European dishes but have been forgotten as people have moved away from the land and come to rely more on food shops. Elderberries don't keep very well, once harvested, so are not popular among growers and shopkeepers. Elderberries contain potent antiviral active constituents, which can relieve the symptoms of colds and flu. They are also effective against herpes and other immune deficiency disorders.

Interactions: elderberries may antagonise immunosuppressant drugs and have an additive effect on chemotherapy, caffeine, diuretics, and laxatives.

Garlic

This aromatic herb has an old reputation for keeping vampires away! It's an idea that may actually be based on fact, not fiction: in Central Asia, and central-eastern Europe—including Transylvania—a rare variety of the disease porphyria was once relatively common. Porphyria is an inherited blood disorder that causes the body to produce less haemoglobin, the protein in red blood cells that carries oxygen. Symptoms are sometimes called attacks and include extreme paleness, anaemia, and a complete intolerance to sunlight. Relief from some of the these may have been found in garlic's medicinal properties. So, hanging out a bunch of garlic for the "vampire" may have started as an offer of help and relief, not banishment.

Garlic (*Allium sativum*) is a plant so ancient that no one is really sure of its origins. It is known to have been cultivated in Egypt and Mesopotamia before 2000 BCE. It had semi-divine status in the ancient world and was called upon in the swearing of oaths.

Garlic contains vitamin C, B1, B6, calcium, phosphorous, potassium, iron, selenium, zinc, flavonoids, mucilage, sulphur compounds, and volatile oils. It is antimicrobial, cardioprotective, diaphoretic, expectorant, hypoglycaemic, hypotensive, and cholesterol-lowering.

Now one of the world's most popular herbs, both as food and medicine, garlic is a warming and drying herb. It is also one of the most effective natural antimicrobials, stimulating the production of white blood cells and acting against a wide range of bacteria, fungi, parasites, and viruses, and it is a first-line treatment for infectious disease. It works directly on infections and infestations in the digestive tract, including candida, dysentery, typhoid, threadworm, and tapeworm, and because it contains a volatile oil that is mostly excreted through the lungs, it is also an excellent remedy for respiratory disorders and infections such as bronchitis, influenza, and whooping cough. The oil is also active against tuberculosis, helping to open the airways and get rid of mucus, which also makes it useful for asthma. It may also reduce the virulence of virus infections such as HIV and Covid.

Externally, it can be used for fungal infections such as athlete's foot and ringworm.

One of the most popular modern uses for garlic is in dealing with cardiovascular disease. It helps reduce blood fat and cholesterol levels. Garlic is also an excellent anticoagulant, decreasing the tendency of the blood to clot. It prevents the formation of fat deposits on artery walls (atheroma) and reduces hardening of the arteries (arteriosclerosis)—changes that are accelerated by smoking and eating a diet high in saturated fats and sugar.

Over time, garlic also helps lower blood pressure significantly.

Garlic also has an ability to suppress the formation of cancer cells and enhance the immune system's ability to slow the spread of malignant tumours.

Contraindications and interactions: garlic can cause gastric irritation and should not be used if there is acute stomach inflammation, ulceration, or acid reflux. It should not be used within ten days of surgery or with blood-thinning medication (anticoagulants). It may potentiate insulin and hypoglycaemic drugs, and it may enhance the effects of cholesterol-lowering drugs (statins).

Ginger

Ginger (*Zingiber officinale*) is native to the tropical forests of Southeast Asia and has been used as a food and medicine for well over 3000 years. The fresh root resembles deer's antlers, and the Latin name *Zingiber* is thought to come from the Sanskrit word *singabera*, meaning "horn-shaped".

Ginger adds warmth and a woody-lemony flavour to cooked dishes. It makes an excellent addition to marinades and dressings, and is a key ingredient in many pickles, preserves, chutneys, cakes, biscuits, and breads.

It is rich in volatile oils, resins, starch, amino acids, phenols, vitamin C and B6, magnesium, potassium, and copper.

Ginger is antioxidant, anti-inflammatory, antispasmodic, carminative, antiseptic, rubefacient, anticoagulant, and cholesterol-lowering. For centuries, ginger has been used to ease rheumatic complaints, and modern research has confirmed its anti-inflammatory effect, and it can be used in detox protocols. It is a diffuse stimulant (as opposed to cayenne being a central stimulant), increasing peripheral circulation, which is beneficial for cold hands and feet, Raynaud's syndrome, and to lower blood pressure by creating more internal space. Ginger makes a warming drink that helps improve the flow of digestive juices and is a stimulating tonic for the digestive system. It also protects the liver and reduces nausea, cramping and wind. It is an excellent remedy for any sickness related to motion, pregnancy, and chemotherapy.

Taken as a hot drink with food, it can also be used as an aid to slimming, because it enhances the thermic effect of food, reducing the feelings of hunger, as well as giving a sense of fullness. It is always best taken with food as high doses can be abrasive and cause heartburn.

Ginger is used as an adjunct to cancer treatment because it inhibits proliferation of cancer cells and enhances the effect of radiotherapy.

It is also effective in topical applications for inflamed joints, bursitis, and muscle sprains.

Contraindications and interactions: use with caution in case of stomach problems, gallstones, kidney disease, and bleeding disorders. Avoid before operations as it may have an additive effect on anticoagulants. It may also interact with diabetes medication, high blood pressure drugs, and sedatives. Ginger may increase the absorption of all drugs.

Grapefruit

Grapefruit (Citrus paradisi) is a powerful detoxifier, helping rid the body of harmful microbes and aiding tissue repair. Acting on the digestive system and the liver, its detoxifying action combined with a strong growth-inhibiting effect on bacteria, fungi, parasites, and viruses, means that grapefruit can be beneficial in immunodeficiency, as well as for colds and flu.

Grapefruit contains a wealth of protective active constituents and antioxidants, including vitamin A, C, folate, potassium, bitter principles, flavonoids, citric and phenolic acids, lycopene, fibre, pectin, and saccharides.

It is anti-allergic, antimicrobial, antioxidant, anti-cancer, detoxifying, cholesterol-lowering, and a digestive and immune stimulant. It enhances immunity and wound healing, and may also inhibit tumour growth.

Although citrus fruits are generally best avoided if you suffer from autoimmune disorders, there is evidence that grapefruit improves some inflammatory conditions.

It is also an effective pick-me-up when stress depletes energy reserves. The bitter principles aid digestion and help you get the most out of the food you eat, and it boosts fat metabolism, making it a popular weight-loss food, especially as it is also low in calories and high in fibre. The soluble fibre in grapefruit also helps lower blood cholesterol and other blood fats by binding with them and promoting their excretion from the body. This makes it useful in the treatment of cardiovascular disease and gallstones. By improving detox and digestion, grapefruit can also be used to relieve constipation, and in reducing kidney stones.

Grapefruit seed extract, known as Citricidal, is a natural, broad-spectrum antibiotic, and grapefruit oil is a powerful astringent and antiseptic that can be used to cleanse oily skin and be a gentle treatment for acne and other skin conditions.

Contraindications and interactions: grapefruit may interact with some prescribed medication.

Onion

The onion (*Allium cepa*), as we know it, is a domesticated cousin of wild onions from Central Asia, Turkmenistan, and Iran. The use of onion as a food and medicine can be traced as far back as 5000 BC. Ancient Egyptians viewed its spherical shape and concentric rings as symbols of eternal life and, according to Pliny the Elder (AD 23–79), ancient Romans used onions for eye problems and to heal anything from mouth ulcers and toothache to dog bites, diarrhoea, and back ache.

Onion contains some vitamin C, soluble fibre, sulphur compounds, polyphenols, flavonoids, volatile oils, and phytosterols.

It is expectorant, diuretic, carminative, antispasmodic, hypoglycaemic, anti-asthmatic, anticoagulant, hypotensive, cholesterol-lowering, antioxidant, antifungal, anti-mutagenic, anthelmintic, antiseptic, and antibiotic.

The onion is a useful remedy against arthritis and gout, and is a natural antibiotic useful for all kinds of internal and external infections, especially coughs, colds, and fevers. Onion also helps lower blood fat, blood cholesterol, and blood sugar. It is useful in cardiovascular disease as it helps lower blood pressure and decreases the formation of blood clots and arteriosclerosis.

Helicobacter pylori, which is thought to be responsible for gastritis and stomach ulcers, is inhibited by onion, and it may also protect against stomach cancer by decreasing the conversion of nitrates to nitrites in the stomach. Onion syrup is a useful remedy for colds and cough.

Contraindications and interactions: onions may cause indigestion in those with gastrointestinal disorders. They may interfere with blood sugar medication.

Parsley

Parsley's reputation as a medicinal herb can be traced back as far as the first century AD. The ancient Greeks used to crown their victors with parsley garlands, and it has been used over the centuries as a diuretic, tonic, and digestive remedy.

Parsley *(Petroselinum crispum)* has a gentle, rather neutral, but very characteristic taste and smell. It is one of the most widely used of all herbs.

It is rich in vitamin A and C, and also in iron, calcium, magnesium, and manganese, volatile oil, coumarins, and flavonoids.

It is antioxidant, diuretic, spasmolytic, carminative, antiseptic, expectorant, antirheumatic, sedative, anti-inflammatory, hypotensive, hypoglycaemic, and blood pressure-lowering.

Parsley is a particularly good source of dietary iron, because its vitamin C content helps the iron to be absorbed from the digestive tract. Both the leaves and seeds can be used for their medicinal action, with seeds being the strongest.

As a diuretic, parsley can be used to remove excess water in heart disease, and it can also be used to treat problems of the urinary tract, and to dissolve and pass kidney- and bladder stones.

As a digestive remedy, it will ease wind and colic, and assist in the digestion of protein. It can be used to treat anaemia and arthritis, and also to encourage menstruation and to stimulate milk flow in nursing mothers while also relieving colic and griping in the baby.

It is a very useful tonic during convalescence.

Contraindications and interactions: excessive contact may cause skin reactions. Use with caution during kidney disease. May interact with serotonin medication.

Peppermint

Peppermint (*Mentha piperita*) is a fragrant aromatic herb with an uplifting quality. It is well known for its digestive properties, and it was already cultivated by the ancient Egyptians, and used by Greek and Roman cooks as a flavouring for sauces and wines.

It has been valued over the centuries as a soothing and pleasant aid to digestion, and is mentioned in pharmacopoeias dating back to the thirteenth century.

The active constituents include volatile oils (menthol), tannins, bitter principle, rosmarinic and caffeic acids, gums, resins, carotenes, vitamin E, and methyl-salicylates.

It is anti-emetic, anti-inflammatory, antimicrobial, choleretic, diaphoretic, expectorant, anti-tussive, antiseptic, locally analgesic, and a cooling remedy with a relaxing effect on muscle tension.

Peppermint can be used to relieve indigestion, wind, colic, nausea, and diarrhoea. It has an established reputation in the management of stomach ulcers and can also be of benefit in cases of Crohn's disease and ulcerative colitis.

Peppermint tea is a good substitute for tea and coffee, as well as a soothing remedy for colds and flu, and as an inhalation it can relieve catarrh and ease breathing. It is also a powerful antiseptic, and peppermint oil has a local anaesthetic effect that can be a useful first-aid remedy for toothache.

Crushed fresh peppermint leaves can be applied locally to relieve pain, including headaches, and a peppermint bath can be used to relieve rheumatic and muscle pains.

Peppermint oil is also used to lower blood pressure (as a calcium channel blocker).

Peppermint is also a good remedy for nausea and sickness.

Contraindications and interactions: high doses of the essential oil can cause irritation, and the oil should not be applied to broken skin, nor used in pregnancy or by breastfeeding mothers. Use peppermint with caution in case of gallbladder obstruction, hiatus hernia, and liver disease.

Peppermint oil should not be used if you are on medication for high blood pressure as it may increase the effect and lower your blood pressure too much. It may also increase the effects of immunosuppressant medication (cyclosporin).

Potato

The potato (*Solanum tuberosum*) is a starchy protein food native to the Americas and a member of the nightshade family, Solanaceae. It is believed to originate from southern Peru and northwest Bolivia around Lake Titicaca where potatoes were first cultivated 7000–10,000 years ago.

Potatoes were introduced to Europe by the Spanish in the sixteenth century, and today they are a staple food all over the world and an integral part of many people's diets.

They are high in complex carbohydrates, and their amino acid composition is very close to that of human protein. They are also high in soluble fibre, vitamin B6, C, and K.

The potato is antioxidant, energy-boosting, and helps strengthen immunity. It lowers blood-fat levels, improves tissue oxygenation, promotes a healthy nervous system, and helps the body absorb and use other nutrients and alleviate stomach ulcers, digestive and malabsorption disorders.

For most benefit, eat potatoes in their skins. Hot potato water and raw potato juice are traditional remedies for arthritis and gout.

Contraindications: green potatoes contain glycoalkaloids that are toxic to humans.

Turmeric

Turmeric (*Curcuma longa*) is related to ginger and shares some of the same qualities. The name may derive from the Latin words *terra merita*, meaning "merit of the earth". It is native to tropical Asia and has been valued in Chinese and Ayurvedic medicine for centuries as a remedy for stomach and liver problems, for inflammation, and to treat wounds and tumours.

It was first brought to Europe as a cheaper alternative to saffron (*Crocus sativus*). But while saffron and turmeric do tint foods a similar golden colour, their taste, aroma, and medicinal qualities are distinctly different.

Turmeric has the quality of fire without burning, and it is stimulating, cleansing, and disinfectant.

It contains high levels of curcumin, as well as plant sterols, resins, volatile oils, vitamin C, B3, B6, magnesium, manganese, potassium, copper, iron, zinc, and omega oils.

Curcumin is considered to be the most active constituent—a powerful antioxidant and anti-inflammatory, capable of protecting cells against free radical damage. It has been shown to be more effective than non-steroidal anti-inflammatory drugs (NSAIDs) in dampening inflammation after surgery.

Turmeric is also anti-carcinogenic and liver-protective, cholesterol-lowering, and anticoagulant. It is known to be a good antiseptic, effective against a variety of fungal and bacterial infections. It may also help inhibit the spread of cancer by destroying mutant cells, and it can enhance the effects of chemotherapy and radiotherapy.

It is used for liver, gallbladder, and digestive problems to relieve wind and protect the stomach lining from ulceration, and for inflammatory bowel disease, indigestion, and ulcerative colitis. It is also useful for arthritic conditions, including tendonitis, bursitis, bruises, sprains, and inflamed joints in general.

Turmeric has a protective effect on the cardiovascular system because it lowers blood fat and cholesterol levels as well as inhibiting blood clot formation.

It is also useful for degenerative diseases such as Alzheimer's, type 2 diabetes, arthritis, and pancreatic problems, and it can help reduce histamine levels and increase the production of cortisone in the body.

Turmeric is also used as an anti-ageing remedy to soften the skin and to ease the symptoms of psoriasis.

Contraindications and interactions: although turmeric is non-toxic, care should be taken in cases of gallbladder obstruction and stomach hyperacidity. Turmeric may also interact with chemotherapeutic drugs, and it can have an additive effect on NSAIDs, anticoagulants, and immunosuppressant drugs.

Remember that turmeric is a strong yellow dye that stains!

CHAPTER 19

Politics and food production

The world as a whole produces enough food to feed every mouth in it. Although it has been falling in recent years, the world's cereal harvest alone (3 billion tonnes in 2022) is capable of feeding more than the earth's present population (8 billion in 2022). The harvest in 2022 would give each person 375 kilos of grain—more than a kilo per day, which I doubt anyone would be able to consume! Add to that 80 million tonnes of pulses—a kilo for every single human being per year. Add to that 1.15 billion metric tons of vegetables and a billion metric tons of fruit, and you get the impression of worldwide abundance of food. And so it should, since most of the earth's landmass is covered in plants.

But the world's system of food production is wasteful: almost 80% of total cereal production goes to the raising of food animals. Power in food production is concentrated increasingly in fewer hands. This concentration of power allows the system to manipulate supply and charge higher prices than may be considered reasonable.

British food and health policies are agreed by government officials in the Department for Environment, Food & Rural Affairs (DEFRA) and the Department of Health and Social Care (DHSC) who take advice from expert advisory committees.

These committees are dominated by scientists and businesspeople. Consumers have very little say, and reports are covered by the Official Secrets Act.

Public health problems are political issues, but nowadays there is apparently little interest in promoting good health. Whole, fresh food is not as profitable to sell as processed food.

Everyone knows that refined carbs are empty calories that provide no nourishment. There are plenty of scientific studies showing their detrimental effect on the health of the nation. Even so, Britain has no effective policy on refined carbohydrates, and the average sugar consumption in Britain is 3 million tonnes per year. That is 44 kilos per person per year! If that sounds like a lot, it is because it is! Some 20% of the total calorie intake is sugar, and two thirds of these worthless calories are consumed in processed foods.

Many middle-aged and old people are in bad health, and many children are also tired and unwell. Child obesity now affects 10% of children aged 4–5, with a further 12% being overweight. At the age of 10–11, 23% are obese and 14% overweight.

Animal breeders acknowledge that unhealthy animals may pass on weakness to the next generation. Since we belong to the animal kingdom, the same must be true for people. In the 1930s, the Scottish teacher, medical doctor, nutritional physiologist, and Nobel Peace Prize winner Sir John Boyd-Orr (1880–1971) wrote: "If children of the three [lower] social groups were reared like young farm stock, giving them a diet below the requirements for health would be financially unsound."

The Child Development Programme at the University of Bristol did a survey in 1984 of 100 families' development over three years. Their report read as follows:

"Although official pronouncements state that the only real nutritional problem in Britain is one of obesity, in fact the Project interviewers' experience has shown that there are many malnourished children in the Project samples, some of whom suffer continual illnesses, which are treated by strong drugs or hospitalisation. In turn, the repeated illnesses can lead to delayed development. Continuously sick children lose their curiosity and desire to learn.

"The brain is still developing in the first two years of life. Most of the children from poor households, and many of the better-off children, were eating a poor diet, high in sugars and low in whole foods. This can lead to retarded brain development after weaning. The children will never reach their full potential.

"We noticed a tremendous amount of minor recurring illness, like diarrhoea and chest infection, that just shouldn't be there. The link between diet and chronic illness in children is a very close one."

That generation of children are now adults and, since the problem is far from solved, they are likely to teach their own children similar dietary habits as they grew up with themselves. Add to that the digital revolution, and the amount of time children spend on their digital devices plus the increasing restraint on their freedom and ability to roam and explore their environment, and you have a recipe for cognitive and physical decline increasing with each generation.

Despite the fact that the medical profession recognises lack of fibre, excess saturated fat, refined carbs, smoking, drinking, drugs, stress, and lack of exercise as major causes of death in Britain, and that poor diet is a major public health problem, the government is still reluctant to recognise that processed food is the single main cause of a large number of diseases. The section of the food manufacturing industry whose profits depend on food made from saturated fats, refined carbs, salt, and additives, spends hundreds of millions of pounds every year in an attempt to persuade us that processed food is good for our health.

The British Medical Association's Board of Science and Education report *Diet, Nutrition and Health* (1986) concludes: "Rather than recommending people to eat less fat, sugar and salt, and more fibre, it would be better to state this advice positively by emphasising the advantages on an increase in consumption of fresh fruit and vegetables, wholemeal and other bread, nuts and cereals generally."

The key findings from the BMA's most recent report, updated in 2021, state that:

- In the UK 63% of the adult population are overweight, and 27% are obese.
- 20% of children are obese by the time they reach Year 6.
- Obesity-related diseases cost the NHS in excess of £6bn per year and are calculated to impact wider society to the tune of £27bn per year.
- By 2050, overweight and obesity will cost the NHS an estimated £9.7bn per year, with societal costs of £49.9bn.
- 26% of Year 6 children in the most deprived areas are obese, compared with 11% in the least deprived.

Source: bma.org.uk

In a world where a child dies of starvation every two seconds, an agricultural system designed mainly to feed the meat habit of the rich is indefensible. Yet it continues, because we continue to support it.

Hunger is a social disease caused by the unjust, inefficient, and wasteful production of food. The average meat consumption per person in India is only 6.5 kg per year, or 8% of the average consumption in the UK, which was 80 kg per year in 2021. The average British housecat eats 100 kg of meat per year, which is four times more than an Indian family of four (26 kg per year). The average person in the world consumed around 43 kg of meat in 2014, ranging from over 100 kg each in the US, the UK, and Australia, to only 6.5 kg in India.

The world now produces more than three times as much meat as it did fifty years ago. In 2018, around 340 million tonnes were produced. That corresponds to 80 billion animals being slaughtered every year for their meat. Add to that the 800 million tonnes of milk being produced each year—more than double the amount fifty years ago.

Hidden in those figures is the life lived by each animal, and the food they ate. The quantity of animal feed required to produce one kilogram of meat, eggs, or dairy products is thought-provoking:

For every kilogram edible output,

- Beef cattle eat 25 kg of food
- Sheep and lambs eat 15 kg
- Pigs eat 6.4 kg of food per kilo of pork
- Poultry eat 3.3 kg
- Egg-laying hens eat 2.3 kg
- Dairy cows eat 0.7 kg of food per litre of milk they produce.

Livestock takes up nearly 80% of global agricultural land, yet produces less than 20% of the world's calories.

The world's farm animal population is enormous!

These figures are from 2016:

1.5 billion cattle (up 44% from 1966)
1.0 billion pigs (up 92% from 1966)
1.3 billion sheep
22.7 billion chickens (up from 4.4 billion in 1966)
0.3 billion turkeys.

These are animals raised with the sole purpose of serving as human food.

This makes a total of 26.8 billion farm animals, over three times more than humans on the planet. Livestock make up 62% of the world's mammal biomass; humans account for 34%; and wild mammals only 4%! A decline of an estimated 85%. Add to that the world's poultry biomass (71%), which is more than twice that of wild birds (29%), and it becomes clear that in biomass terms wild mammals and birds are just a fraction of humans and our livestock.

Global animal feed consumption is estimated to be over 6 billion tonnes per year, including a third of all cereal production. The animal feed industry has a $400 billion annual turnover.

The average person in the world consumes approximately 675 kg of food per year. Multiply that by the 8 billion of us that now (2023) share this planet, and you get 5.4 billion tonnes of food needed to feed the human race. This figure is smaller than the amount of food we give to livestock before we eat them! So it could be said that it would be much more cost-effective to literally cut out the middleman and eat the plant foods we produce directly.

That is precisely what a Danish doctor and food scientist did during the food crisis of the First World War (1914–18) when food was becoming scarce. Dr Mikkel Hindhede (1862–1945) was in charge of feeding the nation during the war, and he had the bright idea of selling Denmark's livestock to the Germans and putting the whole Danish nation on a plant-based diet. The result was that there was food enough for everyone in Denmark while in Germany hunger and scarcity was rife. The Germans had more food per capita but a larger share was used for animal production, and famine was widespread in 1918.

According to Dr Hindhede's calculations, the change may have prevented 6300 deaths in the war, and an added bonus was a fall in many different lifestyle diseases, while the death rate also sank to the lowest number ever. To the question whether meat is an appropriate food in times of need, he said: "Meat is the last requirement to be met. If the people must wait until pigs and cattle have sufficient food, they will die of starvation one year before they can get an abundance of meat."

Currently, the livestock population (236 million) in the UK consumes enough grain (20 million tonnes) and soya beans (2.5 million tonnes) to feed over five times the entire human population (68 million). To put it in perspective, the amount of wheat used to feed animals is equivalent to 10.7 billion loaves of bread, and the amount of oats could be used to make 5.8 billion bowls of porridge. Sheep and cattle also occupy 12.6 million hectares of grassland, eating an estimated 90 million tonnes of grass. Some of the land could be used to grow vegetables for people, and some could be set aside for wildlife.

It is hard to grasp how wasteful a meat-based diet really is: by passing plant foods through livestock before we eat the calories ourselves, we end up producing just 10% of the calories to feed human mouths that would be available if we ate the plant foods directly.

To supply one omnivore food for a year requires 3.25 acres.
To supply one vegetarian requires 0.5 acres.
To supply one vegan requires only 0.17 acres.
To supply one cow with food for a year requires 3 acres.

In other words, a given acreage can feed twenty times as many people eating a plant-based diet as it could feeding a cow or a human on a meat-based diet.

In addition to being an obvious and avoidable cause of world starvation, the current intensive farming system, geared to serving a meat-eating population, also infiltrates our lives in other ways: by-products from slaughterhouses are found everywhere—in polo mints and wine gums, for example!

Countless species of plants are near extinction because of overgrazing and spraying. Since 1945, the UK has lost over 95% of flower meadows, 50% of ancient woodlands, 40% of heathlands, and 50% of fens and valleys. In the same period 224,000 miles of hedgerows have been removed to accommodate modern farming equipment and practices.

In the UK, 70% of land is devoted to agriculture. Worldwide, half of all habitable land is used for agriculture, and of this 77% is used for livestock, either directly for grazing or indirectly to grow crops for animal feed.

Around one third of global greenhouse gas emissions come from agriculture. Approximately 70 litres of water per day per head of livestock are needed for cleaning and cooling. A study from Sheffield University in 2020 concluded that only about 3–5% of UK water is used in people's homes, 5% is used by industry to provide goods and services, and the remaining 90% is used in agriculture. In Ethiopia, the situation is similar, with 6% of their water used in households and 94% by agriculture.

Current total population of farm animals in the UK (2022)

Sheep	15,000,000
Cattle and calves	5,000,000
Pigs	4,000,000
Rabbits	1,000,000
Goats	108,000
Deer	30,000
Chickens	117,000,000
Turkeys	11,000,000
Duck and geese	11,000,000
Total	164,138,000

The global production of fish and seafood has quadrupled over the past fifty years. This has put pressure on fish stocks. Overfishing means that fish are caught at a faster rate than they can reproduce and sustain population levels. This problem has led to the invention of aquaculture, or fish and seafood farming.

The annual worldwide catch of fish from the wild is 95 million tonnes per year. This figure has remained relatively constant since the 1990s, while global fish farming has grown rapidly to over 100 million tonnes per year in 2020.

Modern trawler fishing causes deliberate, or incidental annul deaths of hundreds of thousands of seals, dolphins, porpoises, and birds. And fish farms pollute their local environment. For every tonne of farmed fish, 0.75 tonnes of solid waste (faeces and unconsumed food) is discharged into seas and rivers.

Global lobster production reached 200 million tonnes in 2020. Lobsters are kept in recycled sea water in tray storage systems for up to five years, mainly to supply live lobsters to restaurants.

> "Consumers are also citizens. You have a voice. Nothing will change until politicians are sure that there are votes in good food and good health."
>
> Geoffrey Cannon, *The Politics of Food* (1987)

This is the heart of the matter. Until we all realise that not only do our daily choices affect our own health and that of our family, future generations, friends and neighbours, but our choices also affect the health of our ecosystems and environments.

Choices become habits, and habits are hard to change unless you find new and better habits to replace them with when you realise the detrimental effects of bad habits.

Luckily, many people are waking up to this simple truth: nature knows best, and there is more joy in connecting with nature and all its inhabitants than there could ever be in dominating, enslaving and killing plants, people, and other animals.

The more simply you live, the easier it is to be healthy. When you look at food, work out where it came from and what it must have taken for it to land in your possession. What goes into creating a packet of crisps? A pint of milk? A leg of lamb? A lettuce? Or a nettle?

REFERENCES

Bartram, T. (1998). *Bartram's encyclopedia of herbal medicine*. London. Robinson Publishing Ltd.

British Herbal Medicine Association Scientific Committee. (1983). *British Herbal Pharmacopoeia*. Cowling, West Yorkshire. The British Herbal Medicine Association.

Büning, F. and Hambly, P. (1993). *Herbalism*. London. Headway.

Chaitow, L. (2008). *Naturopathic physical medicine*. Philadelphia. Churchill Livingstone.

Chevallier, A. (1993). *Herbal first aid*. Christchurch. Amberwood Publishing Ltd.

Department of Health (1991). *Dietary reference values—a guide*. London. HMSO.

Duke, J. (2008). *The green pharmacy guide to healing foods: proven natural remedies to treat and prevent more than 80 common health common*. United States. Rodale.

Fieldhouse, P. (1996). *Food and nutrition—customs and culture (2nd edition)*. Cheltenham. Stanley Thornes.

Food Standards Agency (2002). *McCance and Widdowson's the composition of foods (6th summary edition)*. Cambridge. Royal Society of Chemistry.

Garrow, JS., James, WPT. and Ralph, A. (editors). (2000). *Human nutrition and dietetics (10th edition)*. London. Churchill Livingstone.

Oxford Geissler, C. and Powers, H. (2017). *Human nutrition (13th edition)*. Oxford. Oxford University Press.

Grieve, M. (1931). *A modern herbal*. London. Jonathan Cape Ltd.

Griggs, B. (1981). *Green pharmacy—a history of herbal medicine*. London. Jill Norman & Hobhouse Ltd.

Hambly, F. (2004). *Herbal medicine for children*. Rochester. Amberwood Publishing Ltd.

Harrod Buhner, S. (2012). *Herbal antibiotics*. North Adams, MA. Storey Publishing.

Hartvig, K. (2012). *Eat to boost your immunity*. London. Duncan Baird Publishers.

Hartvig, K. (2004). *The healthy diet calorie counter*. London. Duncan Baird Publishers.

Hartvig, K. (2016). *Healing berries*. London. Watkins.

Hartvig, K. (2016). *Healing spices*. London. Watkins.

Henderson, RK. (2000). *Neighbourhood forager*. Totness, Devon. Chelsea Green Publishing.

Hoffmann, D. (2003). *Medical herbalism: the science and practice of herbal medicine*. Vermont. Healing Arts Press.

Khalsa, DS. (2003). *Food as medicine*. New York. Atria Books.

Kew, Royal Botanic Gardens. (2016). *The gardener's companion to medicinal plants*. London. Quarto Publishing plc.

Lindlahr, H. (1983). *Natural therapeutics, volume III: dietetics*. Saffron Walden. The CW Daniels Company.

Lust, J. (1974). *The herb book*. New York. Bantam Books.

Marciano, Dr M. and Vizniak, Dr N. *Evidence Informed Botanical Medicine*. 2nd edition. (2015). Canada. Professional Health Systems Inc.

Mabey, R. (1988). *The complete new herbal*. London. Gaia Books Ltd.

Menzies-Trull, C. (2022). *Herbal Medicine, Keys to Physiomedicalism*. Newcastle. Faculty of Physiomedical Herbal Medicine [Publications].

Mességué, M. (1979). *Health secrets of plants and herbs*. London. Collins.

Mills, S. (1985). *The dictionary of modern herbalism*. Wellingborough. Thorsons Publishers Ltd.

Mills, S. and Bone, K. (2000). *Principles and practice of phytotherapy*. London. Churchill Livingstone.

Pizzorno, JE. and Murray, MT. (2013). *Textbook of natural medicine (fourth edition)*. St. Louis. Elsevier.

Ralph, A. and Tassel, M. (2020). *Native healers*. London. Aeon Books.

Robbins, J. (1987). *Diet for a new America*. Walpole. Stillpoint Publishing.

Rogers, C. (1995). *The women's guide to herbal medicine*. London. Hamish Hamilton Ltd.

Rowley, N. and Hartvig, K. (2000). *Energy foods.* London. Duncan Baird Publishers.

Shaw, N. (1998). *The complete illustrated guide to herbs—a simple guide to using herbs for healing.* London. Element Books Ltd.

Walsh, S. (2003). *Plant based nutrition and health.* St Leonards-on-Sea. The Vegan Society.

Hickson, M. and Smith, S. (editors). (2018). *Advanced nutrition and dietetics in nutrition support.* Oxford. Wiley Blackwell.

INTERNET SOURCES

Botanical.com: Mrs Grieves, A Modern Herbal, online copy: https://www.
botanical.com/botanical/mgmh/comindxg.html (accessed December
2022–March 2023)

British Nutrition Foundation. The Science of fat: https://www.nutrition.
org.uk/healthy-sustainable-diets/fat/?level=Health%20professional#
intakesandrecommendations (accessed December 2022–January 2023)

Cardwell, G., Bornman, JF., James, AP., Black, LJ. A review of mushrooms as
a potential source of dietary vitamin D. National Library of Medicine:
https://www.ncbi.nlm.nih.gov/pmc/articles/PMC6213178/ (accessed
January 2023)

Coeliac Disease Foundation: https://celiac.org/gluten-free-living/what-is-
gluten/ (accessed December 2022)

Delimaris, I., PubMed Central: Adverse Effects Associated with Protein Intake
above the Recommended Dietary Allowance for Adults: https://www.
ncbi.nlm.nih.gov/pmc/articles/PMC4045293/ (accessed 5 December
2022)

European Medicines Agency Monographs: https://www.ema.europa.eu/
en/search/search/field_ema_web_categories%253Aname_field/
Herbal?search_api_views_fulltext=monographs (accessed December
2022–March 2023)

Gröber, U. Magnesium and drugs. National Library of Medicine: https://www.ncbi.nlm.nih.gov/pmc/articles/PMC6539869/(accessed January 2023)

Heart UK: the ultimate cholesterol lowering plan: https://www.heartuk.org.uk/downloads/factsheets/uclp-fact-sheet-oct2019-150dpi.pdf (accessed January 2023)

Japelt, RB. and Jakobsen, J. Vitamin D in plants: a review oof occurrence, analysis, and biosynthesis. National Library of Medicine: https://www.ncbi.nlm.nih.gov/pmc/articles/PMC3651966/ (accessed January 2023)

Kew Science Medicinal Plant Names Services—https://mpns.science.kew.org (accessed December 2022–March 2023)

Lewis, RW and Lentfer JW: The vitamin A content of polar bear liver: range and variability. Comparative Biochemistry and Physiology. ScienceDirect: https://www.sciencedirect.com/science/article/abs/pii/0010406X67907827 (accessed January 2023)

McDougall, JD. Lessons from the past, directions for the future: the WW1 startch solution for Denmark. The McDougall Newsletter. Dr. McDougall's Health & Medical Center: https://www.drmcdougall.com/misc/2012nl/jul/lessons.htm (accessed January 2023)

National Research Council (US) Committee on Diet and Health. Trace elements. National Library of Medicine: https://www.ncbi.nlm.nih.gov/books/NBK218751/ (accessed January 2023)

Nielsen, AG and Metcalfe, NH. Mikkel Hindhede (1862–1945): a pioneering nutritionist. PubMed: https://pubmed.ncbi.nlm.nih.gov/27566234/ (accessed January 2023)

Office for Health Improvement & Disparities: Official Statistics: Obesity profile: short statistical commentary July 2022: https://www.gov.uk/government/statistics/obesity-profile-update-july-2022/obesity-profile-short-statistical-commentary-july-2022 (accessed January 2023)

Plants for a Future (PFAF) monographs: https://pfaf.org/user/Default.aspx (accessed December 2022–March 2023)

Revilla, MKF, and Titchenal, A. University of Hawaii: https://pressbooks-dev.oer.hawaii.edu/humannutrition/ (accessed December 2022)

Skoglund, E. and Sandberg, AS. Phytate. Science Direct : https://www.sciencedirect.com/topics/food-science/phytate (accessed January 2023)

Sommerfield, M. Trans unsaturated fatty acids in natural products and processed foods. National Library of Medicine: https://pubmed.ncbi.nlm.nih.gov/6356151/ (accessed December 2022)

Wikipedia on Gluten: https://en.wikipedia.org/wiki/Gluten (accessed December 2022)

Wikipedia on Palmitic acid: https://en.wikipedia.org/wiki/Palmitic_acid (accessed December 2022)

ACKNOWLEDGEMENTS

I would like to express my deep gratitude to all the amazing students, clients, patrons, colleagues, teachers, authors, friends, and family who have contributed, supported, and inspired the writing of this book, in particular—

Alice Livingstone
Alice Rathbone
Allan Hartvig
Anders Hartvig
Andrew Chevalier
Anita Ralph
Ann Richardson
Ann-Britt Fogde Styrbæk
Anna Animelli
Anna Iben Hollensberg
Averil Atkinson
Barbara Wilkinson
Beatrice Tamasova
Bella Beak
Bendle
Birgitte Aksentijevic
Bob Saxton
Booj Beak
Camilla Fayed
Caroline Rogers
Catherine Argence
Cecile Charmetant
Charlotte Charmetant
Charlotte Lueke
Charlotte Yde
CJ Godden
Christine Fynes-Clinton
Christopher Hedley
Daniela Code
David Hoffmann
Egle Koppel
Emilie Rowley
Essie Jain
Frances Hambly
François Salies

Françoise Nassivet
Galit Zadok
Geoffrey Cannon
Gordon Newman
Grete Lyngdorf
Guy Waddell
Hannah Kenward
Hans Knæhus
Hein Zeylstra
Henry Lindlahr
Iain Millership
Jane Ellis
Jennie Weekes
Jesper Hollensberg
Joan Ingle
Joe Goodman
John Morgan
John Robbins
Kathaline Lauge
Kathleen Hanrahan
Kathy Gallagher
Keith Robertson
Kirsten Hansen
Klaus Mitchell
Laura Iturralde
Leon Chaitow
Leona Philips
Linda Heagerty
Linda Wilkinson
Lisa Smith
Louise Hay
Mario Szewiel
Marion Aavik
Mary Canny
Mary Tassel

Mary-Anne Paterson
Maureen Robertson
Maurice Messegué
Maya Morgan
Michael Olden
Mikkel Hindhede
Milena Silvano
Naphia Reggiani
Nic Rowley
Nick Beak
Nick Tuckley
Non Shaw
Oliver Fynes-Clinton
Oliver Rathbone
Pamela Blake-Wilson
Paul Charmetant
Paul Hambly
Peter Firebrace
Peter Goldman
Pia Grönroos
Raphael Charmetant
Rob Ward
Roger Newman-Turner
Sam Halliday
Sandra Goodman
Simon Mills
Sue Mitchener
Tania Pepper
Tessa Hodsdon
Theo Beak
Thomas Bartram
Tracey Chaplin
Tony Carter
Udo Ottow

Kirsten Hartvig,
The Healing Garden
Forest Row 2023

AUTHOR BIOGRAPHY

Kirsten Hartvig ND, MRN, MNIMH, DipPhyt trained at the School of Herbal Medicine, Tunbridge Wells, and the College of Naturopathy and Osteopathy in London. She is an acclaimed nutritionist, medical herbalist, and registered naturopath practising at The Rachel Carson Centre, Emerson College, Forest Row, Sussex.

Kirsten is director of the Healing Garden, a biodynamic physic garden with over 400 species of medicinal plants. It is part of the 22-acre Biodynamic Botanic Garden at Emerson College.

She is the author of 14 books on natural health and writes regular columns and articles for various newsletters and magazines.

Kirsten teaches Nature Cure diploma courses with Dr Nic Rowley. She leads herb walks, and gives talks and workshops on natural health and herbal medicine.

She is herbal medicine and dietetics tutor at the Nordic College of Natural Medicine in Denmark, where she was a government advisor on herbal medicine and part of the Danish Health Authority's Council for Alternative Medicine.

Kirsten has taught nutrition and dietetics at the European School of Osteopathy and the Scottish School of Herbal Medicine Master's degree course, and she developed and taught part of the materia medica programme on the Heartwood Professional Course.

Kirsten developed the YouTube channel Herb Hunters, and the Herbal Medicine Show on UK Health Radio. She is a member of the National Institute of Medical Herbalists and past president of the General Council and Register of Naturopaths.

INDEX

acid
-alkaline diet. *See* alkaline diet
-forming foods, 160
alcohol
    calories in alcoholic drinks, 30
    misuse effect, 29–30
    -related problems, 29–30
    sugar in, 28–29
alkaline ash diet. *See* alkaline diet
alkaline diet, 159–160
alkalising foods, 159–160
allergic syndromes, 38
Allium cepa. See onion
amensalism. *See* antibiosis
amino acids, xii, 32
amylase, 21
anabolic diet, 133–134, 142, 158–159.
    See also diet(s)
anabolism, 133
anaemia, 106–107
angular stomatitis, 74

animal
    -based proteins, 33
    farm, 187
    feed consumption, 184–186
    products, xiii
antagonism. *See* antibiosis
anthocyanins, 165
    in cherries, 169
antibiosis, 139
antioxidants, 123, 165, 167
antioxidant super-berry. *See* blueberry
ascorbic acid. *See* vitamin C
autoimmune disease, 39
avocado, 55, 161–162. *See also* medicinal
    plant foods

Bantu diet, 93
basal metabolic rate (BMR), 18–19
beetroot (*Beta vulgaris*), 163–164.
    See also medicinal plant foods
beriberi, 72, 73

beta
  -blockers, 19
  carotene, 59
  -sitosterols, 55, 162
betacyanin, 163
Beta vulgaris. *See* beetroot
bilberry (*Vaccinium myrtillus*), 164–165.
      See also medicinal plant foods
binge eating, 17
biotin. *See* vitamin B7
blueberry (*Vaccinium corymbosum*),
      165–166. *See also* medicinal
      plant foods
BMI. *See* Body Mass Index
BMR. *See* basal metabolic rate
Body Mass Index (BMI), 19–20
borecole. *See* curly kale
bran fibre, 25
Brassica oleracea acephala. *See* curly kale
brazil nut, 166–168. *See also* medicinal
      plant foods

calcium, 89, 92, 94. *See also* mineral(s)
  absorption and excretion, 92–93
  Bantu diet, 93
  deficiency, 93–94
  hypercalcemia, 94
  osteoporosis, 93–94
  rickets, 93
  supplements, 90
  toxicity, 94
calories, 11, 13, 131
  adjustments, 20
  in alcoholic drinks, 30
  and appetite, 14
  and balance, 13
  basal metabolic rate, 18–19
binge eating, 17
Body Mass Index, 19–20
  conversion values, 131
  empty-calorie diet, 14–15
  fat cells, dieting, and weight
      management, 16
  obesity and eating disorders,
      16–17
  optimum calorie-intake tables, 20

  quality, 15–16
  required, 17
  sustainable weight loss, 17
capsaicin, 169
Capsicum annuum. *See* cayenne pepper
Capsicum frutescens. *See* chilli pepper
carbohydrate, 21
  alcohol misuse effect, 29–30
  digestion, 21
  disaccharides, 22–24
  extrinsic sugars, 23
  fermentation, 22
  Glycaemic Index, 27–28
  intrinsic sugars, 23
  loading, 27
  monosaccharides, 22–24
  non-milk extrinsic sugars, 23
  polysaccharides, 24–26
  proportions in healthy diet, 132
  raw cane sugar, 22
  refined, 182
  refined sugar, 22
  simple sugars, 22–24
  sources of, 21
  sources of complex, 158
  sugar in alcohol, 28–29
cardiovascular risk factors,
      managing, 51
carnitine, 55
Carnival ritual, 149
carotenoids, 59. *See also* vitamin A
castanea. *See* brazil nut
catabolic diet, 133–134, 141–142, 144.
      See also diet(s)
  grading, 145–146
catabolism, 133
cayenne pepper (*Capsicum annuum*),
      168–169. *See also* medicinal
      plant foods
cherry, 169–170. *See also* medicinal
      plant foods
child
  health, 182–183
  obesity, 182
chilli pepper (*Capsicum frutescens*), 168.
      See also medicinal plant foods

chlorine, 100–102. *See also* mineral(s)
chlorophyll, 55
cholecalciferol (D3), 62
cholesterol, 45
    foods with, 47
    foods with high, 52–53
    to lower, 51, 53–54
    -lowering diet, 52–53
    -lowering herbs and foods, 54–55
    reducing foods, 46
chromium, 115. *See also* trace
        elements
    deficiency, 116
    level in food, 116
chylomicrons, 49
Citricidal, 176
Citrus paradisi. See grapefruit
cleavers (*Galium aparine*), 154
    recipes, 154–155
cobalamin. *See* vitamin B12
cobalt, 117. *See also* trace elements
coeliac disease, 39
conjunctivitis, 74
convalescence, 157
copper, 114. *See also* trace elements
    absorption,
    deficiency, 114–115
    level in food, 115
    toxicity, 115
cream nut. *See* brazil nut
cretinism, 118
cud, 45
Curcuma longa. See turmeric
curcumin, 180
curly kale (*Brassica oleracea acephala*),
        170–171. *See also* medicinal
        plant foods

dandelion (*Taraxacum officinalis*),
        171–172. *See also* medicinal
        plant foods
deficiency, 9
DEFRA. *See* Department for
        Environment, Food &
        Rural Affairs
dehydration, 5–6

Department for Environment, Food &
        Rural Affairs (DEFRA), 181
Department of Health and Social Care
        (DHSC), 181
detox-fast, 151
detox herbs, 153
    cleavers, 154–155
    nettle, 153–154
DHSC. *See* Department of Health and
        Social Care
diet(s), 143
    alkalising foods, 159–160
    anabolic diets, 158–159
    catabolic diets, 144–146
    convalescence, 157
    detox herbs, 153–155
    elimination diets, 155
    fasting, 146–153
    healing crisis, 155–157
    in naturopathic treatment, 133
    slimming diet, 144
dietary
    deficiency, 9
    fat guidelines, 48
    recommendations, 7–8
Dietary Reference Values (DRVs),
        7, 23
diet, healthy, 132, 137
    balancing act, 141–142
    eating for health, 137–139
    ketogenic diet, 140–141
    naturopathic diet, 141–142
    paleo diet, 138
    plant-based foods, 137–138
    potatoes, 138
    symbiosis vs. antibiosis, 139–140
digestion
    carbohydrates, 21
    fat, 49–50
    protein, 36–37
disaccharides, 22–24
disease, 128
    autoimmune disease, 39
    coeliac disease, 39
    fat, 50–51
    overcoming, 135

diuretics, 96
doxorubicin, 74
DRVs. *See* Dietary Reference Values
dyslipidaemia, 140–141

EARs. *See* Estimated Average
        Requirements
eating
    binge, 17
    disorders, 17
    for health, 137–139
edible vegetable oils, 49
EDTA. *See* ethylenediaminetetra-acetate
EFA. *See* essential fatty acids
eicosapentaeonoic (EPA), 50
elder (*Sambucus nigra*), 172–173. *See also*
        medicinal plant foods
elimination diets, 155. *See also* diet(s)
energy, 3
    calorie, 11–12
    provided by macronutrients, 11
EPA. *See* eicosapentaeonoic
ergocalciferol (D2), 62
erucic acid, 49
essential and non-essential, 32
essential fatty acids (EFA), 43
Estimated Average Requirements
        (EARs), 8, 31
ethylenediaminetetra-acetate (EDTA),
        109
European blueberry. *See* bilberry

farm animal population, 187
fasting, 146. *See also* diet(s)
    aims, 146–147
    Carnival ritual, 149
    detox-fast, 151
    effects of, 148–149
    guidelines, 151–153
    lean season, 149–151
    Lent, 149–150
    points to consider before, 147–148
    spring detox, 149–150, 152
fat(s), 12, 41
    absorption and digestion, 49–50
    cholesterol and lipoproteins, 45–48

cholesterol-lowering herbs and
        foods, 54–55
choosing cholesterol-lowering diet,
        52–53
chylomicrons, 49
dietary fat guidelines, 48
and disease, 50–51
fatty acids, 41, 44
in food, 48–49
guidelines, 48
lifestyle research, 52
to lower cholesterol, 53–54
lowering cholesterol, 51
managing cardiovascular risk
        factors, 51
monounsaturated fatty acids, 42
polyunsaturated fatty acids, 42–43,
        50
proportions in healthy diet, 132
saturated fatty acids, 41–42
tackling modifiable risk factors, 51
trans fats, 44–45
unsaturated fats, 44
fat-soluble vitamins, 59
    vitamin A, 57, 59–62
    vitamin D, 57, 62–66
    vitamin E, 67–68
    vitamin K, 69–70
fatty acids, 41
fermentation, 22
ferritin, 108
fibre, 24–25
fish farming, 187
flavonoids, 170–171
fluoride, 112. *See also* trace elements
fluorosis, 112
folate. *See* vitamin B9
folic acid. *See* vitamin B9
food, xi. *See also* medicinal plant foods
    abundance and inefficiencies, 181
    acid-forming foods, 160
    alkalising foods, 159–160
    choices, 184
    with cholesterol, 47, 52–53
    cholesterol-lowering herbs and
        foods, 46, 54–55

for communal activities, xv
global production and
    distribution, 181
junk food, 133
plant-based, 137–138
processed food world, 182
production, 181
role in lives and health, xv–xvi
waste, 139

Galium aparine. See cleavers
garlic (*Allium sativum*), 55, 173–174.
        See also medicinal plant foods
general adaptation syndrome, 134
GI. *See* Glycaemic Index
ginger (*Zingiber officinale*), 54,
        174–175. *See also* medicinal
        plant foods
global food production and
        distribution, 181
glucagon, 37
Glucose Tolerance Factor (GTF), 116
glucosinolates, 170
gluten, 38
    -related disorders, 39
Glycaemic Index (GI), 27–28
goiter, 117
grapefruit (*Citrus paradisi*), 175–176.
        See also medicinal plant foods
GTF. *See* Glucose Tolerance Factor

haemoglobin, 105
haemorrhagic disease of the newborn
        (HDN), 69
HDLs. *See* high-density lipoproteins
HDN. *See* haemorrhagic disease of the
        newborn
healing crises, 135, 155
    features of, 156
    ketosis, 156
    symptoms of, 146, 155–156
health
    and nutritional assessment, 135
    -protective micronutrients, 25
Helicobacter pylori, 177
herbivores, 140

hexaphosphate. *See* phytate
high-density lipoproteins (HDLs),
        45, 46
high-protein diets, 38
hydrogenation, 44
hypercalcaemia, 65
hypercalcemia, 94
hyperthyroidism, 119
hyponatremia, 6
hypophosphatemia, 97, 98

idiopathic haemochromatosis, 106
illness, 128–129
insoluble fibre, 25
intensive farming system, 186
intrinsic sugars, 23
iodine, 118. *See also* trace elements
    cretinism, 118
    deficiency, 118–119
    hyperthyroidism, 119
    level in food, 119
    radioactive, 118
    toxicity, 119
IP6. *See* phytate
iron, 104. *See also* trace elements
    absorption, 105–106
    anaemia, 106–107
    in body, 105
    deficiency, 106–107
    ferritin, 108
    forms, 105
    haemoglobin, 105
    milligrams per 100 grams of
        food, 108
    supplements, 90
    toxicity, 107–108

junk food, 133

ketogenic diet, 140–141
ketosis, 156

LDLs. *See* low-density lipoproteins
lean season, 149–151
Lent, 149–150
linoleic acid, 43

linolenic acid, 43
lipoprotein (a) (LPa), 45
lipoproteins, 45–46
livestock agriculture, 184–185
low-density lipoproteins (LDLs), 43, 45
Lower Reference Nutrient Intakes
    (LRNIs), 8
LPa. *See* lipoprotein (a)
LRNIs. *See* Lower Reference Nutrient
    Intakes

macronutrients, energy provided by, 11
magenta tongue, 74
magnesium, 95. *See also* mineral(s)
    deficiency, 95–96
    toxicity, 96
manganese, 120. *See also* trace elements
    deficiency, 120
    level in food, 121
    toxicity, 120–121
ME. *See* myalgic encephalomyelitis
meat
    -based diet, 186
    consumption, 184
medicinal plant foods, 161
    avocado, 161–162
    beetroot, 163–164
    bilberry, 164–165
    blueberry, 165–166
    brazil nut, 166–168
    cayenne pepper, 168–169
    cherry, 169–170
    curly kale, 170–171
    dandelion, 171–172
    elderflowers and elderberries,
        172–173
    garlic, 173–174
    ginger, 174–175
    grapefruit, 175–176
    onion, 176–177
    parsley, 177–178
    peppermint, 178–179
    potato, 179
    turmeric, 179–180
melatonin, 169–170
menaquinone (K2), 69. See also
    vitamin K

Mentha piperita. See peppermint
micronutrients, 30
milk extrinsic sugars, 23
mineral(s), 3, 89. *See also* trace elements
    -absorbing enhancers, x
    absorption of, 90–91
    calcium, 89, 92–94
    chlorine, 100–102
    functions of, 91
    magnesium, 95–96
    major, 92
    phosphorus, 97–98
    potassium, 99–100
    salt, 100–102
    sodium, 100–102
    sulphur, 103
molybdenum, 121. *See also* trace elements
    deficiency, 121–122
    level in food, 122
    toxicity, 122
monosaccharides, 22–24
monounsaturated fatty acids
    (MUFA), 42
MUFA. *See* monounsaturated fatty
    acids
myalgic encephalomyelitis (ME), 163
myristic acid, 42
myrtillus, 164

National Weight Control Registry
    (NWCR), 143
naturopathic health principles, 127
    disease, 128
    illness, 128–129
    nutritional considerations, 129–130
    vital force, 127–128
naturopathy, 135
    diet for health and healing, 141–142
nettle (*Urtica dioica*), 153
    tea, 154
neural tube defects, 82
niacin, 55. *See* vitamin B3
non-milk extrinsic sugars, 23
nonsteroidal anti-inflammatory drugs
    (NSAIDs), 180
NSAIDs. *See* nonsteroidal
    anti-inflammatory drugs

nutrients, xi
  basic, 3
  energy by macronutrients, 11
nutrition
  assessment, 131–132
  intake guidelines, 7–8
  orthodox, 7
  policy, impact and challenges
    of, 183
nutritional assessment, health and, 135
NWCR. *See* National Weight Control
    Registry

obesity, 16
  child, 182
olive oil, 49
omega-6 fatty acids, 43
onion (*Allium cepa*), 176–177. *See also*
    medicinal plant foods
orthodox nutrition, 7
osteoporosis, 93–94

paleo diet, xiii, 138
palmitic acid, 42
pantothenate. *See* vitamin B5
para nut. *See* brazil nut
parasites, 139, 140
parasitism, 139
parsley (*Petroselinum crispum*), 177–178.
    See also medicinal plant foods
peasants' cabbage. *See* curly kale
pellagra, 75–76
peppermint (*Mentha piperita*), 178–179.
    See also medicinal plant foods
pernicious anaemia, 84
Petroselinum crispum. *See* parsley
Peyer's patches, 37
pH, 163
phenothiazines, 74
phosphorus, 97. *See also* mineral(s)
  deficiency, 97
  hypophosphatemia, 97, 98
  toxicity, 98
photosynthesis, xi, 21
phylloquinone (K1), 69. *See also*
    vitamin K
phytate, ix–x, 25–26

phytic acid. *See* phytate
phytochemicals, 170
plant-based
  foods, 137–138
  proteins, 33
polycythaemia, 117
polyphosphates, 109
polysaccharides, 24
  insoluble fibre, 25
  phytate, 25–26
  resistant starch, 26
  soluble fibre, 24–25
polyunsaturated fatty acids (PUFA),
    42, 50
  function of, 43
porphyria, 173
potassium, 99. *See also* mineral(s)
  deficiency, 99
  toxicity, 99–100
potato (*Solanum tuberosum*), 138,
    179. *See also* medicinal
    plant foods
PPIs. *See* proton pump inhibitors
predation, 140
processed food world, 182
protein, xi–xii, 3, 31
  absorption and processing, 37–38
  amino acids, 32
  animal-based, 33
  calories from, 34–36
  diets with high-, 38
  digestion, 36–37
  essential and non-essential amino
    acids, 32
  gluten, 38–39
  plant-based, 33
  proportions in healthy diet, 132
  quality of animal and plant, 33
  requirements, 34
  role in nutrition, 31
  semi-essential amino acids, 32
  sources of, 158
proton pump inhibitors (PPIs), 96
public health and nutrition, 182
PUFA. *See* polyunsaturated fatty acids
purines, 38
pyridoxine. *See also* vitamin B6

radioactive iodine, 118
rape seed oil, 49
raw cane sugar, 22
RDA. *See* Recommended
    Dietary Allowance
RDI. *See* Recommended Dietary or
    Daily Intakes
Recommended Dietary Allowance
    (RDA), 7
Recommended Dietary or Daily
    Intakes (RDI), 7
Reference Nutrient Intakes (RNIs), 8
refined
    carbs, 182
    sugar, 22
resistant starch, 26
retinols, 59. *See also* vitamin A
riboflavin. *See* vitamin B2
rickets, 62, 93
RNIs. *See* Reference Nutrient Intakes
rumen, 44–45
Rumex crispus. *See* yellow dock root
rumination, 45

Safe Intake, 8
salt, 100–102. *See also* mineral(s)
Sambucus nigra. *See* elder
saturated fatty acids (SFA), 41–42
scavengers, 140
Scoville Units, 168
Scoville, Wilbur, 168
scurvy, 86, 87
seafood farming, 187
selenium, 167, 113. *See also*
    trace elements
    deficiency, 113
    level in food, 114
    toxicity, 167, 113
semi-essential amino acids, 32
sensory stimuli, 16
SFA. *See* saturated fatty acids
simple sugars, 22–24
skin problems, 39
slimming diet, 144. *See also* diet(s)
sodium, 100–102. *See also* mineral(s)
    chloride. *See* salt

Solanum tuberosum. *See* potato
soluble fibre, 24–25
spring detox, 149–150, 152
starch, resistant, 26
stearic acid, 42
steroid hormones, 45
sterols, 171
stimulants, 19, 151, 159
stomatitis, angular, 74
stress
    hormones, 37
    vitamin. *See* vitamin B5
sugar
    in alcohol, 28–29
    intrinsic, 23
    milk extrinsic, 23
    non-milk extrinsic, 23
    raw cane, 22
    refined, 22
    simple, 22–24
sulfonamides, 103
sulphur, 103. *See also* mineral(s)
sustainable weight loss, 17

Taraxacum officinalis. *See* dandelion
TBE virus. *See* tick-borne
    encephalitis virus
thiamin. *See* vitamin B1
tick-borne encephalitis virus
    (TBE virus), 165
tocopherols. *See* vitamin E
tolerable upper limit (TUL), 31
trace elements, 89. *See also* mineral(s)
    chromium, 115–116
    classification, 104
    cobalt, 117
    copper, 114–115
    fluoride, 112
    iodine, 118–119
    iron, 104–108
    manganese, 120–121
    molybdenum, 121–122
    selenium, 113–114
    zinc, 109–111
trans fats, 44–45
tryptophan, 57

TUL. *See* tolerable upper limit
turmeric (*Curcuma longa*), 179–180.
          See also medicinal plant foods

unsaturated fats, 44
Urtica dioica. *See* nettle

Vaccinium corymbosum. *See* blueberry
Vaccinium myrtillus. *See* bilberry
vegetable oils, 43
very-low-lipoproteins (VLDLs), 45
vital force, 127–128
vitamin A, 57, 59
     absorption, 59–60
     deficiency, 60–61
     functions, 60
     level in food, 62
     toxicity, 61
vitamin B1, 71
     beriberi, 72, 73
     deficiency, 72–73
     toxicity, 73
vitamin B2, 73–75
vitamin B3, 57, 75. *See* niacin
     deficiency, 75–76
     pellagra, 75–76
     toxicity, 76
vitamin B5, 77–78
vitamin B6, 78–80
vitamin B7, 80–81
vitamin B9, 82–83
vitamin B12, xii, 83–85
vitamin C, 85
     deficiency, 86
     scurvy, 86, 87
     toxicity, 87
vitamin D, xii, 57, 62–63
     deficiency, 64–65
     hypercalcaemia, 65
     level in food, 66
     in microalgae and edible seaweed, 64
     in mushrooms, 63

photosynthesis, 63–64
     rickets, 62
     toxicity, 65–66
vitamin E, 67
     deficiency, 67–68
     level in food, 68
     toxicity, 68
vitamin H. *See* vitamin B7
vitamin K, 69
     deficiency, 69
     level in food, 70
     toxicity, 70
vitamins, 3, 57
     absorption, 58
     classification of, 57, 58
     fat-soluble, 59
     in food, 58–59
     water-soluble, 71
VLDLs. *See* very-low-lipoproteins

water, 3
     dehydration, 5–6
     hyponatremia, 6
     vital role of, 5
water-soluble vitamins, 71
     vitamin B1, 71
     vitamin B2, 73
     vitamin B3, 57, 75
     vitamin B5, 77
     vitamin B6, 78
     vitamin B7, 80
     vitamin B9, 82
     vitamin B12, 83
     vitamin C, 85

yellow dock root (*Rumex crispus*), 91

zinc, 109. *See also* trace elements
     deficiency, 110
     level in food, 111
     polyphosphates, 109
     toxicity, 111

Printed in the USA
CPSIA information can be obtained
at www.ICGtesting.com
JSHW011944230124
55857JS00012B/67